International Perspectives on Women and HIV

Throughout the world, the threat of HIV/AIDS to women's health has become the focus of increased concern. The Joint United Nations Programme on HIV/AIDS (2004) reports that almost 20 million women and girls are living with HIV globally, accounting for nearly half of all people living with HIV worldwide. Infection rates among women are rising in every region worldwide including high-income countries in which heterosexual intercourse may now be the most common mode of transmission. Although there are many contributing factors to the current trends in HIV, most women who become HIV-infected do not practice "high-risk" behaviour. Women worldwide may individually view themselves as less susceptible than men, and may pay less attention about how HIV is transmitted and how to prevent infection. There are also gender inequalities, stemming from sexual double standards that constrain women's access to care, treatment, and support. This work focuses on international perspectives on women and HIV casting a deliberately wide net addressing the issue of the interaction between HIV and gender in a specific geographic area. Our intention is to provide a forum for innovative manuscripts whose contribution to the literature is found in their unique approach to this interaction and application of empirical investigation to unique problems and/or populations.

This material was published in the *Journal of Human Behavior in the Social Environment*.

Samuel A. MacMaster is Associate Professor at the College of Social Work, University of Tennessee, USA.

Brian E. Bride is Associate Professor at the School of Social Work, University of Georgia, USA.

Cindy L. Davis is Associate Professor at the College of Social Work, University of Tennessee, USA.

International Perspectives on Women and HIV

Edited by Samuel A. MacMaster, Brian E. Bride and Cindy Davis

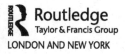

Routledge
Taylor & Francis Group
LONDON AND NEW YORK

First Published 2009 by Routledge
4 Park Square, Milton Park, Abingdon, Oxon OX14 4RN
605 Third Avenue, New York, NY 10017

Routledge is an imprint of the Taylor & Francis Group, an informa business

© 2009 Edited by Samuel A. MacMaster, Brian E. Bride and Cindy Davis

First issued in paperback 2013

Typeset in Times by Value Chain, India

British Library Cataloguing in Publication Data
A catalogue record for this book is available from the British Library

ISBN13: 978-0-415-99837-6 (hbk)
ISBN13: 978-0-415-85228-9 (pbk)

CONTENTS

An Overview

Samuel A. MacMaster
Brian E. Bride
Cindy L. Davis
Lisa Docktor

Throughout the world, the threat of HIV/AIDS to women's health has become the focus of increased concern. The latest report from the Joint United Nations Programme on HIV/AIDS (2004) reports that almost 20 million women and girls globally are living with HIV, accounting for nearly half of all people living with HIV worldwide. Rates are rising, particularly for young women. Since 1985, the percentage of women (aged 15 to 24) living with HIV has risen from 35% to 48%.

Infection rates among women are rising in every region worldwide, including high-income countries in which heterosexual intercourse may now be the most common mode of transmission. From

2001 to 2003, women's prevalence rates increased 5%, making up the largest increase among women in any region of the world. The HIV epidemic's most dramatic increase has been among African-American and Hispanic women, and approximately one-fourth of all North Americans living with HIV are female. In the United States, AIDS is the leading cause of death among African-American women aged 25 to 34. In the Caribbean, girls are almost two times as likely to contract HIV than are boys. In sub-Saharan Africa, 57% of adults with HIV are women, and women aged 15 to 24 are more than three times as likely to become infected than are men of the same age.

Eastern Europe and East Asia have the fastest increase in HIV rates in the world. In East Asia, women make up approximately 22% of adults living with HIV/AIDS. In South and South-East Asia, almost one-fourth of adults and 40% of young people living with AIDS are women.

Although there are many contributing factors to the current trends in HIV, most women who become HIV-infected do not practice "high-risk" behavior. Women worldwide know less than men about how HIV is transmitted and how to prevent infection. There are also gender inequalities, stemming from sexual double standards that constrain women's access to care, treatment, and support.

This book focuses on international perspectives on women and HIV. In soliciting manuscripts for this special issue, we cast a deliberately wide net. It would have been relatively easy to compile manuscripts that addressed the topic through a myopic lens, such as by focusing only on prevention or treatment. We also could have dictated the type of interaction between the three concepts that we were interested in. For example, we could have specified that manuscripts should address the role of gender as a risk factor for contracting HIV or the impact of gender on treatment access. Instead, we left it up to the authors to determine how to address the issue of the interaction between HIV and gender in a specific geographic area and where to place the emphasis. Our intention was to provide a forum for innovative manuscripts with contributions to the literature found in their unique approach to this interaction and application of empirical investigation to unique problems and/or populations.

Sabin and colleagues report on the rapid ethnographic assessment in their work with the Global AIDS Program of the CDC and the Ministry of Health in Honduras. This important piece both provides important information regarding the state of HIV in Honduras and describes the importance of rapid assessments in the continuing battle to maintain surveillance of the spread of HIV.

Burke and colleagues in Australia and Tanzania focus on HIV-positive East African mothers. Their report of a focus group of women provides important suggestions for both HIV prevention and treatment planning. The value of the voice and perspective of women living with the virus and wrestling with these important issues cannot be understated.

While Tanzania and the rest of sub-Saharan Africa are overwhelmed with the rise in HIV rates, South Africa has been a notorious hotspot for HIV transmission among women, where the majority of HIV infections are among young women. Webb-Robbins and colleagues in South Africa report on the results of interventions with caregivers, which aimed to alleviate anxiety depression among participants. The chapter compares results with urban, semi-urban, and rural participants. The results of this study suggest that this may be an important intervention for the well-being of affected individuals both in South Africa and throughout the world.

Within the United States of America, women who contract HIV are increasingly African-American. The next two chapters focus on the prevention needs of two groups of African-American wo-men. Okpaku and colleagues report on an innovative program aimed at increasing treatment access for African-American women who use cocaine, with specific attention to the cultural needs of this population. Smith and colleagues report on the prevention needs among another group of African-American women, those who are involved in the Black Church and the potential resources of the Black Church in providing HIV and other health services.

Webb-Robbins and Ben David provide an interesting and thoughtful overview on the basic economic needs of women, which may need to be addressed prior to the institution of effective HIV programming. Utilizing Maslow's Hierarchy of Needs, the authors suggest that the interconnectedness between economic equilibrium and public health cannot be overlooked.

With its rise economic growth, the country of China is experiencing the most rapidly expanding HIV prevalence rates in the world. Tang reports on the needs for gender-specific interventions that cannot overlook the patriarchal cultural beliefs and inferior social status that many women in China experience. Similar to the previous chapter, Tang reports the need for a larger scope in prevention efforts, fo-cusing on the specific vulnerabilities of women due to the cultural constraints.

Tung and colleagues report on the HIV knowledge of young college women in Taiwan. The results suggest that there was a significant group of individuals who were unaware of HIV and held onto many myths regarding transmission. Clearly there is significant need for prevention interventions for this population.

Continuing the theme of rapid social change and related HIV prevention needs, Humble and Bride report on another hotspot for HIV infection, the country of Russia. Specifically, the authors report on the needs of emerging HIV risk populations in Russia and the role of feminism in the development of gender appropriate interventions.

The chapter by Doshi and Gandhi provides an overview of work and needs in India for HIV prevention among women in that country. The authors report on the status of women and the impact on HIV prevention. Again the reader is provided a cultural context within which HIV behavioral risks exist and the broader social issues that impact the choices that women are able to make.

The need for cultural specific interventions is continued in the last article. Ellis and colleagues report the need for culturally grounded HIV prevention for Latina adolescents in border areas between the United States of America and Mexico. The article makes the case for specificity in developing gender- and cultural-specific programming.

This book is an addition to the literature that depicts both the breadth of the relationship between gender and HIV as well as how closely these phenomena are linked. Gender plays a key role in the prevention and transmission of HIV. Early in the epidemic, HIV infection and AIDS were rarely diagnosed in women. Today, the HIV/AIDS epidemic represents a growing and persistent health threat to women around the globe. (UNAIDS, UNFPA, & UNIFEM, 2004). Women now represent half of all adults living with HIV/AIDS, with the percentage as high as 60% among young women between the age of 15 and 24. As compared to that of men, the picture is much grimmer for women. Women are at risk for sexually transmitted HIV for several reasons, including biologic vulnerability, lack of recognition of their partners' risk factors, power, inequality, gender norms, and the inability to negotiate safer sex practices within the relationship. Some women may be unaware of their male partners' risk for HIV infection and feel powerless to insist on safe sex practices. HIV prevention is particularly challenging for women, given the inequality to negotiate safe-sex practices. Some women are not able to insist on condom use owing to inequality in the relationship and/or out of fear that their partners will physically abuse them or leave them (Foreman, 2003; Gupta and Weiss, 1993; Suarez-Al-Adam, Raffealli & O'Leary, 2000). According to the gender and power theory, women's risks of HIV infection is heavily influenced by socioeconomic factors, power imbalances within relationships, and gender-specific cultural norms.

It is essential to consider these factors when implementing HIV-prevention programs for women around the globe.

These twelve chapters provide innovative conceptual models, research findings, and recommendations to the practice field that are applied to a diverse body of women affected by HIV. As individual works, they are important; when taken together under this rubric, the true nature of the multi-layered and interconnected relationship between these issues begins to emerge. It is the untangling of this relationship that the editors believe holds great promise for continued research that develops a better understanding of these phenomena and ultimately improves the lives of women and girls touched by HIV.

REFERENCES

Foreman, F. E. (2003). African American college women: Constructing a hierarchy of sexual arrangements. *AIDS Care, 15*(4), 493–504.

Gupta, G., & Weiss, E. (1993). *Women and AIDS: Developing a new health strategy (Policy Series, No. 1)*. Washington, DC: International Center for Research on Women.

Joint United Nations Program on HIV/AIDS (UNAIDS), United Nations Population Fund (UNFPA), & United Nations Development Fund for Women (UNIFEM). (2004). *Women and HIV/AIDS: Confronting the crisis*. Geneva: Author.

Suarez-Al-Adam, M., Raffealli, M., & O'Leary, A. (2000). Influence of abuse and partner hyper-masculinity on the sexual behavior of Latinas. *AIDS Education and Prevention, 12*, 263–274.

UNAIDS (Joint United Nations Programme on HIV/AIDS). (2004). *2004 Report Women and AIDS: Confronting the Crisis*. Geneva, UNAIDS/UNFPA/UNIFEM.

Rapid Ethnographic Assessment of HIV/AIDS among Garífuna Communities in Honduras: Informing HIV Surveillance among Garífuna Women

Miriam Sabin
George Luber
Keith Sabin
Mayte Paredes
Edgar Monterroso

Garífuna, an Afro-Caribbean ethnic group living on the north coast of Honduras, has been noted to have one of the highest HIV prevalence (8.4%) rates in Central America (Sierra et al., 1999). Garífuna women of child-bearing age are at particularly high risk for becoming HIV-infected, raising the specter of increased maternal to child transmission of HIV (Trujillo, Paredes, & Sierra, 1998). Garífuna women are burdened with issues affecting HIV transmission such as negotiating safe sex, low levels of HIV prevention knowledge (Tercero, Arana, & Miranda, 2002), and poor access in some regions to HIV testing or treatment for HIV-infected individuals (Stansbury

& Sierra, 2004; Tercero et al.). In addition to HIV, Garífuna women, and women in general in Honduras, face such structural issues as poverty, intimate partner violence, low literacy and poor access to comprehensive healthcare (Tercero et al.; UNAIDS/UNFPA/UNIFEM, 2005). All these factors likely contribute to high HIV prevalence and poor HIV-related health outcomes among Garífuna women.

Owing to their high risk of acquiring HIV, Garífuna in Honduras are considered a focus population for HIV prevention activities by the Honduras Ministry of Health and its partners (CDC & World Bank, 2003). Garífuna women require effective public health and social service interventions to lessen the burden of HIV in their communities. These interventions should be informed by the stakeholders. Surveys linking HIV prevalence and HIV-related risk behaviors over time, including sexually transmitted infection (STI) rates, should be used to monitor and evaluate the effectiveness and impact of the interventions developed according to *Second Generation Surveillance* guidelines (UNAIDS & WHO, 2000). *Second Generation Surveillance* often employs repeated behavioral surveys that can include biomarkers for either or both HIV and selected STIs. The surveys are commonly referred to as *Behavioral Surveillance Survey Plus Biomarkers* (BSS+; Family Health International, 2000). Such behavioral surveillance surveys also provide insight into the most effective way to target HIV prevention interventions. Planning for care and treatment of HIV-infected individuals uses estimates and projections of HIV transmission rates derived from STI and HIV seroprevalence over time in combination with behavioral factors (CDC, 2005).

In this article, we briefly describe the Garífuna and provide an overview of the HIV epidemic in Honduras and among Garífuna at the time of this assessment. We will then discuss how rapid ethnographic assessment (REA; Scrimshaw & Hurtado, 1987), a formative, qualitative methodology, was used to inform a BSS+ survey of HIV/AIDS among Garífuna communities on the north coast of Honduras. The purpose of this assessment is to guide effective public health surveillance and ultimately improve HIV interventions through on-going monitoring and evaluation.

GARÍFUNA

Garífuna origins can be traced back to 1675 when a ship carrying West African slaves destined for the Americas shipwrecked and the would-be slaves escaped (Gonzalez, 1988). Over time, Garífuna migrated throughout the Caribbean and Central America, forming, to some extent, family units with the local Amerindian population and maintaining many West African cultural traditions (Gonzalez). Such distinct ethnic groups that differ from the surrounding local populations require sensitive attention to ethnomedical, non- "Western-tradition" health beliefs, treatment-seeking, and social structure to adequately validate any survey methodology and its questionnaires (Herman & Bentley, 1993).

Garífuna utilize a range of traditional healers for health care needs (Barrett, 1995; Coe & Anderson, 1996; Blanchard & Bean, 2001). The term *witchcraft* is used, and witches, or *buiyes*, perform and lead community ceremonies closed to outsiders, often incorporating rituals, dances, drumming, trances to contact the dead: at times these ceremonies are conducted to seek revenge (Gonzalez, 1988). Sick individuals often visit traditional healers first for non-biomedical interventions to assist with illnesses, including AIDS-related illnesses (Tercero et al., 2002). Surveys examining treatment-seeking behavior in the informal (ethnomedical) sector should carefully assess any effects healers and this treatment-seeking may have on a given health condition (Scrimshaw & Hurtado, 1987).

Health-seeking behaviors among indigenous groups in resource-poor settings are often constrained by socioeconomic factors that must be adequately assessed prior to survey implementation. Farmer (1999) notes that biomedical interventions are expensive by local standards and there is often little to no access for such care; indigenous people of low socioeconomic status may seek traditional healers because they are often cheaper and more readily available. This may be the case among Garífuna communities where access to biomedical care for HIV/AIDS is limited primarily to the regional center La Ceiba, a city on the north coast, a day's travel (with mandatory overnight) from the more remote Garífuna communities.

Status of Garífuna Women

Garífuna women live in a society in which the majority of men migrate seasonally to the United States or other locations for work and thus spend significant periods of time away from the community (Tercero et al., 2002). Because the primary male partner of a Garífuna woman is often away, Garífuna women are in charge of household affairs (Tercero et al.). Garífuna women reportedly have sufficient social status to be heads of household, share income-related decisions, and have multiple sex partners (Tercero et al.). However, a qualitative HIV risk factor survey for the Honduras Ministry of Health in 1999 reported widespread intimate partner violence (IPV) by Garífuna men against Garífuna women. Garífuna women's status may not be linked to full social access. Further review of Garífuna women's actual social status and power within the family and society is needed (Stansbury & Sierra, 2004). Myths that reflect an exoticism to Garífuna culture may interfere with accurately assessing gender interactions important to HIV transmission. Any quantitative survey, such as the BSS+, needs to carefully delineate the extent to which these common beliefs may mis-inform survey practices among Garífuna and prospectively correct them prior to survey implementation.

Economic progress among Garífuna has been difficult since Hurricane Mitch devastated Honduras in 1998 (Inter-American Development Bank, 1999). Of Garífuna who remain in Honduras, many men earn a living from wage work in San Pedro Sula, the largest North Coast city, in textile (*maquila*) factories or by fishing/conch diving (Stansbury & Sierra, 2004). A subsequent coconut blight that struck the North Coast devastated the majority of coconut trees in the region; Garífuna struggle to find sufficient quantities of palm fronds for housing, community structures, food, and coconuts for making bread, puddings, and shells to make carved jewelry that support their income (Canadian Interdevelopment Agency, 2002).

Status of Women in Honduras

Honduran women, in particular those of lower socioeconomic status, are faced with similar social and economic barriers as Garífuna women face owing, in general, to poor access to credit, technology, training, equal salaries, and land (Canadian Interdevelopment Agency, 2002). As with Garífuna, it is estimated that 8 of 10 women experience IPV in Honduras (U.S. Department of State, IWRAW). Honduras passed the *Law Against Domestic Violence* in 1997 (National Congress of the Government of Honduras, 1997) to increase the penalties for domestic violence crimes. Physical and sexual violence are reportedly widespread; the UN Population Fund (2000) estimates that 8 of 10 Honduran women experience such violence in their lifetimes. The same proportion of working women (8 of 10) is living under the poverty line. In 1998, the national per capita income per woman was 47.3% of men's national per capita income (Canadian Interdevelopment Agency). According to the *UN World's Women* report the percentage of deliveries attended by skilled health staff in 1996 was 47%; the maternal mortality ratio was 220 per 100,000 live births for 1998. Illiteracy rates are similar for Honduran women (27.2%) and men (27.1%); the majority of Hondurans complete only elementary school (85.4%) (Perfil Ambiental de Honduras, 1997). Overall, women in Honduras confront multiple problems of daily living to survive.

Overview of HIV/AIDS in Honduras

Honduras, with 17% of the population of Central America, at the time of this assessment, had 44% of Central America's reported AIDS cases, in part owing to a stronger AIDS case reporting system than its neighboring countries (UNAIDS, 2004). An estimated 63,000 people are living with HIV/AIDS (PLWHA) in Honduras, and there is a national HIV prevalence of 1.9% (UNAIDS, 2005), however, the Global Fund estimates that 30–50% of HIV cases are not reported (Global Fund, 2004). There has also been a steady increase in the prevalence of women with AIDS as compared with men with AIDS (UNAIDS), with a one to five percent range of HIV prevalence among antenatal clinic (ANC; clinics for pregnant women) surveillance sites. The AIDS cumulative incident case rate in 1997 in the Department of Atlantida, on the northern coast of Honduras, and an area where the majority of Garífuna live, was reported to be 357.2 per 100,000 (Trujillo, Paredes, & Sierra, 1998).

HIV Prevalence and Related Risk Factors among Garífuna

In 1998, the Honduras MoH conducted a serosurvey (N = 310; Sierra et al., 1999) among high-risk groups in Honduras, including Garífuna. Ten percent of commercial sex workers (CSWs) were HIV-infected; 8% of men having sex with men (MSM) and 7% of male prisoners were HIV-infected. Five percent of 16- to 20-year-olds were HIV-infected. The HIV prevalence rate among Garífuna was found to be comparable, 8.4%. Sixteen percent of Garífuna 16- to 20-year-olds, in comparison to 5% of 16- to 20-year-olds in the general population were HIV-infected. HIV prevalence was relatively evenly distributed among male and female Garífuna (8.5% of males and 8.2% of females, respectively), suggesting the epidemic largely involves heterosexual transmission (Sierra et al.). The 1998 AIDS cumulative incident case rate in the same region was 2,000 per 100,000 (Trujillo et al., 1998) or 18% higher than the population incident rate in Atlantida (357.2

per 100,000; Trujillo et al.). There have been no additional surveys in the past 7 years, and at the time of publication in 2008, these rates may no longer apply.

Stansbury and Sierra (2004) report the *Association El BuenPastor* conducted a Knowledge, Attitudes, Behaviors and Practices survey among Garífuna communities in 2000; findings suggested a knowledge gap in which knowledge of HIV/AIDS was high among participants (90%), but awareness of specific risk factors was low. For example, only 5.5% of participants self-reported that mother to child transmission was a risk (p. 458).

A 2002 REA on the cosmology (Garífuna universe) and behavior around AIDS among Garífuna in North Coast communities with the highest AIDS incidence rates examined Garífuna HIV/AIDS risk perceptions and behaviors (Tercero et al., 2002). In general, the authors suggested high incidence of HIV among Garífuna is largely due to multiple sex partners, migration to and from the United States where migrants are ostensibly becoming infected, use of Traditional Healers instead of Western medicine, and poor access to preventive care and services (p. 2). The results from the qualitative analysis indicated factors involved in the high rate of HIV among Garífuna women included sexual debut in adolescence, little to no condom use, poor knowledge of HIV risk behaviors nor accurate awareness of prevention messages, and gender-power gap issues (such as, ability to negotiate condom use, IPV and drug and alcohol abuse by male partners; p. 31). Pregnant adolescent females may be especially vulnerable to becoming HIV-infected because they tend to have no male partner or husband yet and thus engage in commercial sex work to provide income for themselves and their baby (p. 33). Findings also showed that HIV prevention messages are largely shared within the context of the voluntary counseling and testing session.

These surveys indicate that Garífuna are at high risk for acquiring and transmitting HIV. Overall, their unique risk factors such as migration within major urban centers in Honduras and to and from the United States (Shedlin & Shulman, 2004), the cultural practice of multiple sex partners, transactional sex, minimal reduction of HIV risk-related behaviors (such as little to no condom use), and women's difficulty to negotiate safe sex are reported to be common (Stansbury & Sierra, 2004; Tercero et al., 2002), but no formal behavioral surveillance system is currently in place. Behavioral surveillance integrated with biomarkers could assess behavioral trends over time and provide a more accurate assessment of the true prevalence of HIV among Garífuna.

OBJECTIVE AND METHODS

The objective of this study was to inform the BSS+ study protocol. Study methods were qualitative and based on an REA approach (Scrimshaw & Hurtado, 1987) in which a limited number of narrowly focused study questions are addressed in a time-limited manner. In this case, we used the REA to inform a quantitative study, the BSS+. The REA utilized multiple data collection methods: focus groups, key informant interviews and participant observation.

Literature Search

The literature search was organized into searches of the peer-reviewed literature from the following databases: PubMed (MEDLINE); Sociofile; PsychInfo; Anthropological Index; and Honduras Ministry of Health reports. Other statistics were requested from the Honduras Ministry of Health and GAP/Central America and Panama Office.

Key Informant Interviews

Key informant categories developed prior to travel included Ministry of Health staff; non-governmental organization (NGO) staff working with Garífuna; Garífuna community representatives; health care professionals working in Garífuna communities; and select Garífuna community members, such as health promoters and health clinic workers.

Semi-Structured Interview Guide

A semi-structured interview comprising six domains and containing open-ended questions facilitated standardized discussions across key informant category participants and ensured that study objectives were met. The six domains of the semi-structured interview included (1) community acceptability to conduct the BSS+; (2) response to sensitive questions: sexual behaviors, alcohol and drug use, other HIV/STI risk behaviors; (3) acceptability to collect biomarkers for HIV and STIs; (4) gender-specific concerns and differences; (5) migration; and (6) survey logistics. When a semi-structured interview was not appropriate (impromptu informal meetings), interviews were completely open-ended. Key informant interviews were conducted on an ongoing basis throughout the REA period.

Focus Group Discussions

Prior to the REA, we planned focus groups for the following categories: NGO members; Garífuna community leaders and/or health promoters and providers; and Garífuna community members involved in HIV/AIDS work in their communities. Groups of no more than 90 minutes' duration were led using the semi-structured interview guide and additional probe questions when required to further clarify participant responses. All six domains were queried in all interviews, wherever possible, but not all questions were necessarily included in all interviews. In some instances, questions were dependent on type of respondent, (e.g., health clinic worker or community member). Where appropriate, focus group discussions (FGDs) were taped. Tapes were used to enhance the researchers' notes and were not intended for transcription, which is timely and costly. Oral consent was obtained from FGD participants prior to taping. Typically, participants received drinks (soda), and in one case, a meal (eaten with the researchers) to compensate them for their time.

Site Visits. Site visits were conducted on an ongoing basis to tour prospective Garífuna BSS+ sites, to determine suitability of health clinics as BSS+ survey sites, and to determine local capacity in HIV/AIDS work. Site visits included pre-selected BSS+ sites, as well as Garífuna communities where the researchers had contacts or scheduled visits.

Site Selection, Key Informant and Focus Group Selection. We used a purposive sampling strategy based on place and person from a list of previous contacts, from additional referrals by key informants, and from prior field experience. The Honduras office of the U.S. Peace Corps assisted with contact of health sector Peace Corps volunteers who work, and in most cases, live in Garífuna communities and have the community's trust. Three volunteers facilitated or organized meetings or FGD or assisted with entré into specific Garífuna communities.

REA Study Team. The strongest rapid assessment teams are composed of social scientists trained as observers, who have good listening skills and who know how to facilitate a discussion without leading it (Scrimshaw & Hurtado, 1987). In this case, the study team comprised an anthropologist/epidemiologist and a social worker/social scientist, both with prior ethnographic experience in indigenous Latin American communities. We also enlisted the assistance of a Peace Corps volunteer working at an HIV/AIDS advocacy NGO on the north coast of Honduras with close and trusted ties to the Garífuna communities we needed to visit.

Data Analysis

Data were analyzed following a qualitative content analysis model. We wrote detailed notes from all encounters, and focus groups were audio-taped. We had a daily co-review of meeting notes to elicit convergent (or common) themes and divergent (or discordant) themes across focus group participants and interviews. Data were not divided by different focus group populations or locations because divergent opinions among groups were otherwise negligible and not considered to differ appreciably. Results and recommendations were based on consensus review by investigators.

This REA study protocol was reviewed for human subjects considerations and received a determination of non-research at the CDC.

RESULTS

Sample

In 2 weeks in late 2004, we conducted 17 key informant interviews, 3 FGDs, and 11 site visits to clinics and NGOs and 6 Garífuna communities: La Ceiba, Trujillo (Barrio Cristales), Tela, Triunfo de la Cruz, Tornabe, and La Encenada. The three FGDs, with a total of 30 participants, consisted of a PLWHA advocacy group; community health promoters group; a community leaders group. Seventy-five percent of FGD participants were female (Table 1).

Domain 1: Community Acceptability to Conduct the BSS+ (Table 2)

"People are dying from HIV. It is not rare."

—HIV/AIDS nurse, key informant

Five primary questions were asked in this domain comprising the following areas: (1) severity and importance of HIV/AIDS in Garífuna communities; (2) acceptability of discussing HIV/AIDS; (3) presence

TABLE 1. Characteristics of Focus Group Participants, Honduras, November 2004

	Gender (n)		
	Women	Men	Location
1. Health Committee/Health Promoters from ~10 Garífuna communities	21	0	Tournabe, Garífuna community, North Coast
2. Persons living with HIV/AIDS community-based organization	4	2	San Juan la Encenada, Garífuna community, North Coast
3. Community leaders group	2	1	San Juan la Encenada, Garífuna community, North Coast
Total number of participants:	30		

or absence of status in the community after receiving an HIV-positive diagnosis; (4) types of healers accessed for treatment (i.e., Western-medicine style versus traditional; and (5) behavior change related to HIV-positive diagnosis or due to the problem of HIV in their communities.

Convergent themes in these areas indicated that it is appropriate to discuss a wide range of sexual behaviors as well as alcohol and drug use. Key informants and FGDs did stress that Garífuna will discuss these topics only with persons who have been given approval

TABLE 2. Domain 1: Community Acceptability of Behavioral Surveillance Survey Plus Biomarkers (BSS+), Key informants and Focus Group Participant Themes, November, 2004

Community Acceptability	Convergent Themes	Divergent Themes
1. Severity and importance of HIV/AIDS	Severity and importance recognized	Trujillo region: HIV/AIDS seen as less severe problem
2. Acceptability to discuss HIV/AIDS	HIV/AIDS education and visibility of PLWHA has improved acceptability to discuss the disease	Confidentiality remains a problem
3. Status change after learning HIV-positive status (stigma)	PLWHA are generally considered of the same social standing as community members who are not HIV-positive	Stigma remains a problem in some families
4. Behavior change related to diagnosis	Behavior change not occurring	None

by community leaders or those with established community trust; otherwise false answers may be given on the BSS+ survey.

There was a general understanding of the severity or importance of the epidemic. However, a divergent theme emerged from discussions with key informants in the Trujillo area. In Garífuna communities in Trujillo and its environs (a remote, largely rural location), there may be a difference in perception related to severity and impact of HIV on their communities. Contacts in Trujillo discussed a myth or prevailing belief that there is a governmental conspiracy to portray Garífuna as having high rates of HIV, and therefore these reportedly high rates were believed to be false. There was also the perception that traditional healers (*buyies*) had cures for HIV/AIDS. Despite the regional difference and related different health-seeking behaviors, there was agreement that, in general, Garífuna communities have been exposed to many educational campaigns, programs and capacity building of local health promoters by local NGO's and Ministry of Health workers in community health clinics. Another commonly discussed point was that despite high HIV/AIDS prevalence, awareness was not translating into behavior change. At the time of survey, condoms were reportedly rarely used within communities or not used at all within multiple partner networks. Condoms are available in communities but were reported by several key informants to be largely purchased by foreigners or men from Honduran cities going to Garífuna communities to have sexual relations with local Garífuna women ("male weekenders").

Common myths among the Garífuna such as that persons who look healthy do not have HIV/AIDS, or that youth are too young to have HIV/AIDS (and thus are sought out as sexual partners) or that only CSWs have HIV/AIDS may also influence lack of behavior change. An underlying factor involves economic privation that was indicated to influence decisions to purchase condoms or to engage in CSW, or to enter into sexual relationships to obtain other resources (such as "in style" clothing or electronic appliances). Many Garífuna relationships were reported (by key informants and focus group participants uniformly) to involve women who seek men to provide resources for themselves and their children, but this should not be confused with what is commonly thought of as CSW (direct money-for-sex transactions).

Generally, participants said that discussing HIV as a topic is acceptable among families who have family members with HIV/AIDS and within the community, as well as with friends of the family. Acceptability was reported to vary by individual families. Some health promoters who work with parents of youth with HIV+ diagnoses reported occasional difficulties in engaging these families in treatment owing to denial. Some parents may refuse treatment for their teenage son or daughter. FGD participants and key informants overall concluded that the ability to discuss HIV, especially as it relates to family members, is due to a reduction in stigma-related issues among Garífuna communities. This should not be confused with women's concerns about sharing HIV-positive results with their partners, which appears, among Garífuna, to be related to gender concerns rather than stigma. Stigma appears to be viewed as a community level response to HIV/AIDS.

There was agreement among focus group participants that the social status of an HIV+ individual does not change after receiving a positive diagnosis. Stigma was described as having been a barrier to community acceptance and treatment following diagnosis in years past, but is no longer perceived to be a problem. Another reason given for a lessening of HIV-associated stigma is due to the perceived endemic nature of HIV in Garífuna communities. Few families are not personally affected by HIV, and when both caregivers in a family die, AIDS orphans are taken in by family or other community members. However, focus group participants indicated that stigma still exists in certain families and may be more problematic in the communities in and around Trujillo.

In a focus group discussion with PLWHA who are also community health promoters, mental health status of PLWHA was reportedly another possible barrier affecting treatment-seeking behaviors for HIV. Common responses described by the promoters included feelings of hopelessness, denial, and depression. Respondents suggested that these responses may be moderated by level of adequate access to treatment or to the absence of a cure for HIV.

Domain 2: Response to Sensitive Questions Regarding Sexual Behaviors, Alcohol and Drug Use, and Other HIV/STD Risk Behaviors (Table 3)

"Garífuna are not shy about discussing sexual behaviors."

—Focus group participant

We were told uniformly in all key informant interviews and FGDs that Garífuna are accustomed to hearing about intimate sexual behaviors and talking about HIV risk behaviors (as long as trusted community members were involved in such a study and the discussions took

TABLE 3. Gender-specific Concerns Associated with BSS+ Participation, Key Informant and Focus Group Participant Themes, November 2004

Gender-Specific Concerns	Convergent Themes	Divergent Themes
1. Disclosing HIV sero-status to participant's sexual partner (partner notification)	IPV possible if confidentiality related to HIV sero-status is not upheld	None
2. Disclosing participant's risk behaviors to the participant's sexual partner	IPV possible if sexual behaviors (like commercial sex work) are disclosed to sexual partner	None

place in confidential settings). Youth are also engaged in educational campaigns and create and act in their own plays on HIV and are already exposed to knowledge about HIV transmission.

Ritual cutting was not reported, and few men reportedly have tattoos. Informal injections for medicinal purposes and injection drug use were not reported. When we asked about cocaine use, health promoters reported that cocaine and crack cocaine are used by some individuals in the Garífuna communities.

Domain 3: Collecting Biomarkers

"Garífuna are used to giving blood samples but need incentives to participate."

—Garífuna community leader

Garífuna reported that it is acceptable to collect biomarkers but that venipuncture, rather than finger-stick blood collection, is viewed as less painful and thus preferred. A private space, such as the community health clinic, maximizing confidentiality was viewed as essential to maintaining confidentiality. This is particularly important for women respondents with intimate partner safety concerns.

Domain 4: Gender-specific concerns (Table 3)

"If I ask my man to use a condom, he will think I did something, like prostitution and that I have HIV."

—Focus group participant

Participants indicated that it is possible that IPV directed toward the female could be a consequence of partner notification of HIV status. They also uniformly indicated that sexual risk behaviors on the part of the female respondent, often a part of voluntary counseling and testing for HIV, would be risky if discussed with a male partner. Gender issues with regard to discussing sexual practices and risk-reduction strategies were explored with community key informants and focus group participants. Health promoters/nurses stated that there have been cases of women being injured by partners for this reason. There was agreement that IPV is a problem only if the partner is informed of the woman's status. One community health professional stated that there is no partner notification in her community because she would be "killed" if she notified either the male or female partner of the other's status.

Ability of women to negotiate condom use with partners was explored as an indicator or proxy for individual female control over their lives and to explore risks related to intimate partner violence. Health promoters in a FGD commented that women have little to no negotiating power related to sex and condom use. Two promoters gave specific examples of common male partner statements such as (1) a woman who asks for a condom has engaged in CSW, (2) the woman would appear to have a higher level of education than the male, which is unappealing to the male, (3) there would be a risk of IPV for suggesting condom use, (4) men refuse to wear condoms (men reportedly say their penises are too large and will break the condoms if used), (5) condom use does not feel good, (6) the woman is not at risk for contracting HIV because she is the man's primary partner, and (7) if a woman wishes to use a condom then she must be HIV-positive. Women also stated that they fear losing their primary partner if they insist on condom use, which also affects the family income.

Other themes of the FGDs and key informant interviews suggested Garífuna women may be at risk for contracting HIV owing to not using condoms, having multiple sex partners, CSW (reportedly not common), having sex with the primary partner who has sex with multiple partners and CSWs in the cities or abroad. FGDs indicated that Garífuna are reportedly not monogamous. Unofficial primary relationships or marriages (*union libres*) are common and are based often on the ability of the male and female to provide needed resources for the family and home.

Most respondents agreed that they did not believe there would be any difference between men and women with regard to their willingness to submit to HIV testing and that there was no difference between males and females to seek testing or treatment. This may appear a contrary notion given women's concerns about potential IPV, but FGD participants indicated that women's concerns are mitigated by having a well-trusted provider and confidential clinic setting.

Domain 5: Migration

"June through August when everyone comes home from New York City is the best time to do the survey."

—Health promoter key informant

Migration, both domestic and international, is an important aspect of Garífuna social and economic life. Internal migration to and from the community to urban centers for work is reportedly common for males and females, and international migration primarily to New York City is common among males. We were told uniformly in FGDs and interviews that men return to their communities in June through August. While both men and women leave their communities to seek work, men usually leave for longer periods of time. Participants also reported migration among Garífuna communities to and from Belize, Guatemala, and Honduras.

There was strong consensus among respondents that they believe migrants to be the core transmitters of HIV. Women reported knowing the risks of having sex with their partners who return from long tours abroad but again discussed their difficulty in negotiating safe sex practices. Health promoters and key informants also acknowledged that women have other partners when their primary sex partner is away.

Domain 6: BSS+ Survey Logistics

"Men fish at night and sleep late in the morning. Interview in late afternoon."

—Health promoter key informant

Garífuna men are traditionally fishermen. Fishing generally takes place at night or early morning which is reportedly the best time to receive large catches. Consequently, men sleep in the morning. Migration is such an important factor in the cycle of HIV transmission for these communities, convergent themes indicated the survey should attempt recruiting returning migrants by sampling when they have returned to their communities (i.e., June–August). Nearly every community has a health clinic that can function as confidential and trusted location to conduct the HIV testing and interviews.

Questionnaire-Associated Findings. In addition to answers from the six domains, we received information from key informants that could be used to improve the usefulness of the BSS+ questionnaire, in particular about sexual behavior questions. Garífuna men and women appear to routinely have multiple sex partners. Garífuna women may add a sexual partner when their primary male partner is working in the United States. Men are likely to have additional sex partners when abroad in U.S. urban centers. Some women may exchange sex for resources when working as domestics in San Pedro Sula, an area with high HIV prevalence. In addition, a wide range of sexual activities, considered routine among Garífuna we spoke with, were described, such as MSM, women having sex with women, and high-risk behaviors such as unprotected anal intercourse. Treatment-seeking questions may need revision in the Garífuna questionnaire. For example, we heard from multiple sources that Traditional Healers tell Garífuna that the healers have cured them of AIDS. We also were told that traditional healers were providing incorrect information on HIV/AIDS. We did not collect specific examples of inaccurate information.

Recommendations. Recommendations to BSS+ partners were made in 2004 and included the following: community leader and HIV/AIDS workers' buy-in is essential. Garífuna data collectors are needed. The survey can be conducted in Spanish, but interviewers should speak both Spanish and Garífuna. Incentives must be provided to maximize participation. Private rooms in community health centers are required to engender confidentiality and reduce IPV concerns. Women who have IPV concerns may be more hesitant than others to answer questions truthfully, might conceivably be less willing to consent to HIV testing, and might not accept the offer to receive their HIV testing results. Our results, however, did not yield these issues as likely to happen. The survey should be conducted in June-August when both international and domestic Garífuna populations return to their communities. Finally, the BSS questionnaire should reflect a range of sexual and treatment-seeking behaviors; however the questionnaire should be pilot-tested to ensure readability and to enhance question validity on such questions. In order to enhance truthful answers, participants should be asked questions in a manner that is respectful to the community being surveyed.

DISCUSSION

This REA provided critical details for the development of a stronger Honduras BSS+ protocol; an added asset to this assessment was Garífuna community leaders affirming the importance of assessing HIV-related risk behaviors and seroprevalence of HIV and STI's in their communities. Survey acceptability is contingent on a respectful, collaborative approach with community leaders, on providing incentives, and offering test results in a safe, confidential space. Our initial literature search suggested Garífuna women may have gender-specific risks from participating in the BSS+. Partner notification in high-prevalence settings is sometimes offered as a part of HIV counseling and testing. In this case, if we had not explored women's IPV concerns, partner notification may have been considered, with possibly adverse consequences for some women respondents. FGDs and key informant interviews suggested that women may equally agree to HIV counseling and testing, despite personal IPV concerns; however, this appears to be because the community health providers and individuals are not disclosing HIV positive results to partners.

There is evidence from two prior qualitative studies examining Garífuna HIV-related risk behaviors (Tercero et al., 2002) and conceptions of HIV/AIDS (Stansbury & Sierra, 2004) that gender inequity is a critical risk factor involved in the high HIV prevalence among Garífuna women, especially those of child bearing age. The REA from Tercero et al. (2002) and this REA both elicited the same themes, suggesting greater validity for these results: Women lack the ability to negotiate condom use with their sexual partners. Women interviewed in both studies indicated that requesting their partner use a condom is synonymous with "promiscuity" or that the women must be HIV+ but are not telling the truth to their partner.

Green (2001) studied differences among rates of the same variables used in similar style rapid assessments utilizing mixed qualitative/quantitative methods versus large, national surveys in developing world settings and found that overall, there were no statistically significant differences between the REAs and the large surveys. The only difference was the cost of doing a national survey versus an REA. In addition to informing the BSS+ protocol, using an REA in this context was consistent and able to build upon existing research findings.

In this survey, comments related to condom use suggested that not using condoms may also be associated with HIV-related stigma. Respondents in our REA indicated that people living with HIV/AIDS no longer face social discrimination; on a more intimate level, condom use may be associated with HIV and thus can be stigmatized among sexual partners. It will be important for any future prevention interventions among Garífuna to reframe condom use messages.

In this study, we found Traditional Healers may be sharing incorrect HIV prevention messages; respondents also indicated that some healers tell Garífuna attendees that they are cured or can be cured of HIV. Healers are a well-established health care alternative for many Garífuna (Tercero et al., 2002; Stansbury & Sierra, 2004; Gonzalez, 1987; Blanchard & Bean, 2001; Barrett, 1995), especially if access to biomedical health care is too expensive or hard to reach. It will be important to incorporate treatment-seeking behavior questions in the BSS+ protocol and to develop educational interventions for healers. This would serve the dual purpose of improving accurate information and including healers in HIV activities, rather than marginalizing them.

This REA provided recommendations to the key stakeholders for the BSS+, and many recommendations were added to the BSS+ protocol. Specifically, the protocol did include recommendations from the REA, such as, that the survey will take place in the summer months, as recommended; that Garífuna data collectors will be used; clinics will conduct the testing, local support will be enlisted, the questionnaire will be modified to reflect a range of Garífuna sexual and HIV risk-related behaviors, and the instrument will be pilot-tested with the Garífuna. Since this REA, there has been tremendous regional interest in the need for formative, rapid ethnographic assessment to inform BSS+ surveys. The CDC/GAP Central America and Panama regional office planned other rapid ethnographic assessments to inform other BSS+'s in the region. One such assessment was recently conducted among the Kuna Indians in Panama.

There were several limitations to this rapid ethnographic assessment. This was not a representative sample. Non-random selection of individuals for focus groups, while appropriate for this type of assessment, may have introduced a selection bias. We had time and logistical constraints and were unable to visit all Garífuna communities, and we may have introduced our own personal biases into the data analysis.

There was insufficient time for data transcription, which may have elucidated additional themes; however, this rapid work is in lieu of a more formal qualitative approach that is data- and resource-intensive and time-consuming. Obtaining information on the exact number of health care facilities and services for HIV-positive individuals was beyond the scope of work for this assessment but would be important to consider for BSS+ implementers.

CONCLUSION

Garífuna women have difficulty overcoming economic, material, and social obstacles that may impact their acquiring HIV. The BSS+, with sufficient instrument changes and pilot testing, is the first survey to give a panoramic view of the HIV epidemic and factors contributing to high transmission rates among Garífuna on the North Coast of Honduras. The BSS+ is leading to targeted HIV prevention messages and programs relevant to Garífuna risk-related behaviors and to permit evaluation of the current package of programs. As many factors such as migration and economic disadvantages are not immediately obtainable, accurate prevention strategies based on well-informed, well-executed surveillance are the foundation for lowering HIV and STI transmission rates in this population. Likewise, gender equity of Garífuna women is not a current reality but may be viable as part of an overall prevention strategy among Garífuna. REAs in Garífuna communities informed the BSS+ protocol development and the survey itself. Qualitative methods in unfamiliar contexts are essential for formative study and inform systematic surveys.

REFERENCES

Barrett, B. (1995). Ethnomedical interactions: Health and identity on Nicaragua's Atlantic Coast. *Social Science & Medicine, 40*(12), 1611–1621.

Blanchard, D. S., & Bean, A. (2001). Healing practices of the people of Belize. *Holistic Nursing Practice, 15*(2), 70-78.

Canadian International Development Agency. (2002). Gender profile: Honduras, April, 2002. Retrieved November 23, 2005, from http://www.acdi- cida.gc.ca/cida_ind.nsf/0/b192afe6e51058748525bf80063458e?OpenD...

Centers for Disease Control and Prevention. (2005). Global AIDS Program Surveillance Fact Sheet. Retrieved December 6, 2005, from http://www.cdc.gov/nchstp/od/gap/docs/program_areas/About%20Our%20Work_Surveillance.01.05.pdf

Coe, F. G., & Anderson, G. J. (1996). Screening of medicinal plants used by the Garífuna of Eastern Nicaragua for bioactive compounds. *Journal of Ethnopharmacology, 53*, 29–50.

Family Health International. (2000). Behavioral surveillance surveys BSS: Guidelines for repeated behavioral surveys in populations at risk of HIV. Retrieved December 6, 2005, from http://www.fhi.org/NR/rdonlyres/eefxryoi4dijq64z7l2hda2l6672dvkhjzyqol5i6gv zy3dcpvoue5zgjsqtbl2sdt55dg2faeee3p/bssguidelinesfull.pdf

Farmer, P. (1999). *Infections and inequalities: The modern plagues.* University of California Press.

Gonzalez, N. L. (1988). *Sojourners of the Caribbean: Ethnogenesis and ethnohistory of the Garífuna.* Champaign, IL: University of Illinois Press.

Gonzalez, N. L. (1979). Garífuna settlement in New York: A new frontier. *International Migration Review, 13*(2), 255–263.

Green, E. (2001). Can qualitative research produce reliable quantitative findings? *Field Methods, 13*(1), 3–19.

Herman, E., & Bentley, M. (Eds.). (1993). *Rapid assessment procedures (RAP): To improve the household management of diarrhea.* Boston: International Nutrition Foundation for Developing Countries.

Inter-American Development Bank. (1999). Hurricane Mitch: Women's needs and contributions, Women in Development Program Unit. Washington, DC: Sustainable Development Department Technical Papers Series. Retrieved on December 6, 2005, from http://www.iadb.org/sds/doc/soc%2d115e.rtf

National Congress of the Government of Honduras. (1997). Law against domestic violence, decree 132-97. Retrieved on December 6, 2005, from Harvard Law School http://ns.rds.org.hn/participacion_ciudadana/legislacion/leyes_secundarias/ley_contra_la_violencia_domestica.html

Scrimshaw, S. C. M., & Hurtado, E. (Eds.). (1987). *Rapid assessment procedures for nutrition and primary health care.* Los Angeles: UCLA Latin American Center Publications and the United Nations University.

Shedlin, M. G., & Shulman, L. (2004). Qualitative needs assessment of HIV services among Dominican, Mexican and Central American immigrant populations living in the New York City area. *AIDS Care, 16*(4), 434–445.

Sierra, M., Paredes, C., Pinel, R., Fernandez, J., Mendoza, S., Branson, B., et al. (1999). Seroepidemiologic study of syphillis, hepatitis B and HIV in the Garifuna population of El Triunfo de la Cruz, Bajamar, Sambo Creek and Corozal. In *Report from the Honduras Ministry of Health, Subsecretary for Populations at Risk.* The Department of Control and Prevention of Sexually Transmitted Diseases, AIDS and Tuberculosis. Honduras Ministry of Health, Tegucigalpa, Honduras.

Stansbury, J. P., & Sierra, M. (2004). Risks, stigma and Honduran Garífuna conceptions of HIV/AIDS. *Social Science & Medicine, 59*, 457–471.

Tercero, G., Arana, C., & Miranda, L. (2002). Cosmovision, comportamiento y SIDA: Un estudio de antropologia medica entre los Garifunas (Cosmovision, behavior and AIDS: A study of medical anthropology among the Garifuna) Honduras: Report: Interamerican Development Bank Program on Technical Co-operation, October, 2002.

Trujillo, O. G., Paredes, M., & Sierra, M. (1998). HIV/AIDS: Analysis of the evolution of the epidemic in Honduras. Health Promotion Foundation, National Center for Control and Prevention of AIDS, Ministry of Public Health, Honduras. Honduras Ministry of Health, Tegucigalpa, Honduras.

UNAIDS. (2004). 2004 report on the global HIV/AIDS epidemic: 4th global report. Joint United Nations Programme on HIV/AIDS (UNAIDS), Geneva, Switzerland.

UNAIDS/UNFPA/UNIFEM. (2005). Women and HIV/AIDS: Confronting the crisis (2005). Retrieved on December 6, 2005, from: http://genderandaids.org/downloads/conference/308_filename_women_aids1.pdf

East African Mothers with HIV: Testing, Talking, and Transmission to Children

Jean Burke
Neema Peter Majule
George Ikongo
Michael Burke

Three quarters of HIV-infected women in the world (15 years and over) live in sub-Saharan Africa (an estimated 13.2 million) and outnumber HIV-infected men about 3:2 (UNAIDS, 2006). The AIDS epidemic in East Africa has reached alarming proportions and continues to increase. In the United Republic of Tanzania, the HIV prevalence rate among adults (ages 15–49) is 8.8%, according to

UNAIDS, based on surveillance data for 2003 (UNAIDS, 2004). Women tested in antenatal clinics have an even higher prevalence rate, of 12% (UNICEF, 1999). This corresponds to 1,600,000 adults living with HIV, including 840,000 women and 140,000 children. Thus HIV or AIDS affects every family. Heterosexual intercourse is the predominant means of HIV transmission in sub-Saharan Africa. Mother-to-child transmission (MTCT) is the most common source of HIV transmission to children. It can occur in the womb, during childbirth, or during breastfeeding. Without intervention, there is about a 30% risk that a baby born to an HIV-infected mother will also be HIV-infected (Marseille, Kahn, Mmiro, et al., 1999; Guay, Masoka, Fleming, et al., 1999). A variety of interventions are required to address each of the transmission modes, some specifically.

Strategies to prevent HIV transmission from mother to child in high-income countries include antiretroviral drugs, elective cesarean sections, and avoiding breastfeeding (Mandelbrot, Le Chenadec, Berrebi, et al., 1998). Prevention of mother-to-child transmission of HIV faces special challenges in lower-income countries such as Tanzania. There are higher rates of HIV infection among childbearing women, fewer HIV counseling and testing facilities, limited access to family planning services, universal breastfeeding with little safe alternatives, and a need for practical drug regimes that are affordable and simple (UNAIDS, 2000).

Scientific research has established the feasibility of cost-effective and simple drug interventions to reduce HIV transmission from mothers to children in Africa (Marseille, Kahn, Mmiro, et al., 1999; Guay, Musoka, Fleming, et al., 1999). Pilot projects of the antiretroviral drugs, zidovudine (AZT), and nevirapine have been implemented in African countries, including Tanzania. These drugs have been initially piloted in five hospitals in Tanzania and are now being scaled up throughout the country.

The use of antiretroviral drugs and strategies to prevent HIV transmission from mothers to children relies on women knowing their HIV serostatus through voluntary counseling and testing (VCT) services. Infant feeding options suitable for HIV-positive mothers to use vary according to the individual and community context. In areas of high infant mortality and infectious diseases, breast milk substitutes are not only too expensive but can pose a risk for infant survival. Exclusive breastfeeding, early weaning, and pasteurization of breast milk are all being debated as alternative options to reduce MTCT risk. All require the identification of HIV status of mothers and the provision of information and counseling.

The agencies of the United Nations have presented a four-pronged strategy to reduce HIV transmission to children. The approach involves (1) services to prevent women from becoming infected with HIV, (2) prevention of unintended pregnancies among women who are HIV-infected, (3) use of antiretroviral drugs, safe delivery practices, and infant feeding options to reduce the transmission of HIV from mother to child, and (4) care and support for HIV-positive mothers, their children and families (UNAIDS, 2001).

It needs to be kept in mind that fertility rates are high in Tanzania, with women in rural areas having 6.5 children on average while their urban counterparts have 3.2 children (National Bureau of Statistics [NBS], 1999). The median age of marriage for women is 18.1 years, about 5 years earlier than men (NBS, 1999). Fertility is highly valued in Tanzanian society, and people are considered full adults only when they become mothers or fathers. Proof of fertility is frequently expected prior to marriage. Promiscuity is the expected norm among men, even when married, but not for women. Polygamy of up to four wives is officially allowed within the Islamic religion. Early marriage and age at first sexual intercourse for women correspond with prevalence rates of HIV among young women, which are about double that of young men (UNAIDS, 2000).

CONTEXT

The region of Dodoma is located in the center of Tanzania, with a population of 1.6 million people. Most people in this semi-arid region are farmers and cattle keepers. The predominant tribe is Gogo. A large variety of tribes are represented in the town center. The region as a whole has an annual food deficit of 2 to 3 months. It is classified by the government as one of the four most vulnerable regions to food insecurity owing to the lack of reliable rain (Water Aid, 2000).

The AIDS Control Programme of a faith-based organization situated in Dodoma offers comprehensive services ranging through counseling and testing, community education and training of volunteers, and care and treatment (for opportunistic infections) of people with HIV. Presently, very few pregnant women seek HIV testing and only at the advice of doctors because they have symptoms of AIDS. This program, familiar to the authors, was considering how to expand services to address prevention of HIV transmission to children. Linked to this program is a support group of people living with HIV as well as a self-help group of people living with HIV. Some members of this group are actively open about their HIV status, even teaching others about HIV in public forums.

PROBLEM

The earliest studies on HIV infection have tended to take an epidemiological approach, focusing on biological, individual, or group risk behavior. However, the sociocultural dimensions of the AIDS epidemic are being increasingly recognized in research and interventions. Gender inequality is evident in uneven political and socioeconomic status, double sexual standards, and a lack of decision-making power for women within male-female relations. The vulnerability of women and the resulting range of reproductive health problems are factors that increase the spread of HIV infection in Africa (Awusabo-Asare & Anarfi, 1999: 1). Research can be a channel for voicing experiences and needs (Wadsworth, 1997) and giving women greater visibility (Oakley, 1981).

One of the greatest challenges in controlling the spread of AIDS in Tanzania and other African countries is that the majority of people living with HIV and AIDS do not know it. The themes "It's better to know" and "Breaking the Silence" of international AIDS conferences acknowledge this. The contribution of groups of people living with HIV to care, support, and prevention within the AIDS epidemic has been recognized as essential and in need of strengthening. This has been formalized as the principle of greater involvement of people living with HIV and AIDS (GIPA) (UNAIDS, 2000). Piot states, "People with HIV must play an integral role in HIV prevention and care programs in order for them to be truly effective" (UNAIDS,

2000). People Living with HIV and AIDS (PLHAs) can bring first-hand experience to AIDS action. Their experience is their expertise. The authors recognize that open and active HIV-positive women can offer insights into the challenges and dilemmas that may be faced by women and men seeking to prevent HIV transmission to children in future. Understanding their feelings, experiences, and concerns can inform and guide the development of relevant services.

METHOD

Participants

Six HIV-positive women were interviewed for this study conducted in Dodoma, Tanzania. These women are all active members of groups of people living with AIDS. They are members of a support group that meets monthly with several staff from the local AIDS Control Programme. Most members have been counseled and tested within this program, and they continue to receive counseling and free medical treatment (for opportunistic infections). They are also members of a self-help group, which is a branch of a national network of self-help groups for PLHA. They meet regularly for formal meetings and more often informally for mutual support. Some of the women work voluntarily as counselors and educators.

Design and Procedure

Women were chosen who have known their HIV status for at least a year, were well enough to be interviewed, and were known to be not pregnant at the time. The women had reached a stage where they themselves express an acceptance or peace about their HIV status, have been open with others about their HIV status, and have sought the company of others like them. These are characteristics they have in common with each other. Such a group is not representative of all African HIV-positive women, many of whom do not know they have HIV or hide their knowledge. Interviewing pregnant women was considered outside the scope of this study. However, the selected women were considered to have relevant experiences that they would be able to share and reflect on without major distress. The women were invited to participate by the chair of the self-help group. There were no refusals. Other women were included in a later group meeting which discussed the six women's recommendations.

The main topics explored in the qualitative semi-structured interviews were the women's experiences of voluntary counseling and testing, disclosure of HIV status, caring for their children, and opinions about MTCT of HIV and drugs. Permission to publish the results was given by the National Institute of Medical Research, Tanzania. Feedback of the women's opinions and advice was discussed in a group meeting with them. A focus group of women and men living with HIV more specifically discussed interventions to reduce mother-to-child HIV transmission.

The small sample of this study allows only the women's experiences to be described and issues to be raised on the basis of these experiences. The sample size is inadequate to be the basis for any conclusive statements or results. The stories and insights they share are illustrative of the impact of culture and the social environment on women's behavior in the context of HIV. The women are neither representative nor typical of HIV+ women, who are more likely to be unaware of their HIV status, or to remain silent. Instead these women were highly interested and relatively well-educated about HIV. However, this also meant they were engaged and motivated to discuss the issues.

RESULTS

Knowledge and Choices

Interviews were recorded, transcribed in Swahili and then translated into English for greater ease in analysis. Qualitative thematic analysis combined and compared answers and recommendations. Within interviews, statements about women's experiences were compared with advice given to check validity. Common issues and patterns of concerns emerged from the data.

The six women are a diverse group who range in age from 25 to 52 years. All are mothers who are currently without partners: Three are widows, and three are separated. Two have HIV-infected children. All are primary school-educated. Most run small businesses in the informal sector or have no paid work. The diversity of age, religion, background, and experiences limits the nature of any conclusions drawn from this study. However, their particular contexts and experiences illustrate specific dilemmas facing women and mothers with HIV.

Choosing to Be Tested for HIV. For all the women, knowing their HIV status was beneficial and informed their choices. The women were motivated to be tested for HIV by their own sickness or the sickness or death of their partner, often encouraged by friends, relatives, or the advice of a doctor. They sought testing to address concerns about their own health rather than in relation to childbearing. Even so, their experiences and choices have been affected by the reality of MTCT of HIV. At times their choices have been limited by their own or their partner's sickness and also by not knowing they were living with HIV.

Karol is a 52-year-old single farmer who was tested for HIV at the advice of a doctor. She was worried about her health as she had lost weight and was continuously sick. She found that she was HIV-positive at a time when she was still breastfeeding her child. Karol wonders whether she was infected through a needle injection after childbirth and recalls that she had shivers and fevers a week later, which could correspond to acute infection.

> *"My child was $1\frac{3}{4}$ years of age and I was breastfeeding. I asked if she had got the disease. The doctor said I should wean my child. This was just a secret between my doctor and I ... The father has gone to the village. He is expecting me to die ... I tested my child's blood—it is positive. I haven't told her. She is still young (8 years old)."*

Karol's positive results allowed her to take action to protect her child from further exposure to HIV transmission through breast milk. Unfortunately, her child was already infected. She continues to keep this knowledge about her child's HIV status confidential. Karol believes she has been infected with HIV for 10 years already.

Martina is a 32-year-old woman who is separated from her Muslim husband. She previously had a child with another partner. She felt she had had a good marriage, but her husband's family applied pressure when she didn't have a child. They wanted her husband to get a second wife. This prompted her to consider HIV testing and using condoms.

> *"Before he got another wife, I wanted us to check our health. But he refused. I got very SERIOUS. I asked for us to use the modern way. Let's use condoms. If not, it's better I leave."*

Her discussion about using condoms highlights the double function of condoms as protection from sexual diseases and as contraception and how these may contradict. Her request to use condoms was more likely to be a message to her husband that she was not happy about him getting another wife. This constructs the new wife as a potential health risk.

Despite her apparent lack of decision-making power in the family, Martina went alone to be tested for HIV. She continued to try to negotiate with her husband. He left her and married a much younger woman. She believes he is HIV-infected, but he refuses to be tested.

> *"The counseling was good—to get a choice. I was advised about sex and to put effort into telling my partners. Also to try to use condoms. But I feel worried using them and finding a place to buy them. But then when it came to using them, he (her husband) refused."*

Martina attempted to gain more control over her sexual life. Negotiating the use of condoms was a way to assert her responsibility to protect others and her right to protect herself from further infection from her husband while he was in another sexual relationship. She, however, faced resistance to this. In her case, because of its contraceptive function, the use of condoms could also be perceived as refusal to have another child. Counseling gave her information about options. Her social context restrained these options from becoming real choices. Different outcomes may have been possible if her husband had participated in counseling with her. It is possible that he also is infected with HIV and that HIV may be transmitted to his new wife and new children without his knowledge. Martina herself thought it was impossible that there could be one HIV-positive and one HIV-negative person in a sexually healthy relationship. Therefore she believed her husband was also infected with HIV.

Choosing How to Communicate. All the women thought it better for a husband and wife to be tested together, if possible. In this way, options could become choices. The benefits of testing together were stated to be that they could talk to each other truthfully and with understanding, and have opportunities to love, care, forgive, and be open and free with each other. They would not be able to deceive each other by keeping the test result to themselves. They could discuss and make plans together, such as about their sex life and childbearing.

*"If it happens, it's best to say bad luck, not to say it came from
the woman's side or the man's side and break the marriage. They
need to plan, discuss and love each other- to live this way. It
takes time to be open." (Naomi).*

Naomi missed this chance, as she found out her HIV status only after
her husband died. She would have preferred to be able to talk about
HIV with him, without blaming or placing the responsibility on him
for their infection. Five of the women interviewed stated that they
had been faithful to their sexual partners and had therefore made no
change in sexual behavior once they found out their HIV status.

Madala is a 45-year-old Muslim businesswoman, divorced with two
married children. She had eight other children who had died. She was
initially tested for HIV in hospital without her knowledge or consent.
Two years after hearing her results, she has not yet told her own
children. She plans to do so.

*"I told my mother and brother. My brother told me that he
already knew my results but hadn't told me. It was when I
was tested in the hospital. He'd told me it was typhoid. They
accepted it well. They just looked after me, saying don't carry
the burden. They helped me, showing love and giving hope....
They collected money together for me ... I felt happy. I didn't
worry about being turned away by my family. I was worried if
they had rejected me, how would I live?"*

Ironically, Madala's family knew her HIV results before she did.
Although she feared their rejection, she was surprised by their warmth
and practical help to her.

Sofi is a 25-year-old Muslim widow who sells goods in the informal
sector. Her husband became sick and was anxious about his health.
Sofi recalls that he tried to talk to her about the possibility that he
was sick with AIDS.

*"On the radio they were talking about AIDS. My husband said,
'I need to tell you something. If I said I have AIDS what would
you do?' I said 'OK. I will know that you are positive, but I
will have nothing to do but wait for death.' He said, 'I was only
joking.'"*

Sofi recalls this conversation as an attempt by her husband to talk
about HIV in an indirect way. It appears he wanted to test her possible

response to disclosure of his own results. Since her hypothetical response was to despair, he decided to wait until a later time. When her husband heard an openly HIV-positive person speaking on the radio later, he encouraged Sofi to go and seek counseling with that person. After this, Sofi and her husband were counseled and tested for HIV together.

Choosing to Live with Hope. For three of the women, the initial news of their positive HIV status led them to consider suicide, hence endangering their life. Each considered swallowing poison or medicines. They passed through their times of despair comforted by relatives, spiritual writings, and counseling. Access to counseling was a highly appreciated aspect of knowing about being HIV-positive. Several women spoke passionately about its benefits.

"I will never forget the help I got until the day I die." (Sofi)

"Without the counseling, I'd be in a bad state." (Madala)

"Now I laugh and smile and people ask me why am I laughing!" (Naomi)

"I got comfort—like medicine." (Vivian)

This last metaphor of the effect of counseling being like medical treatment emphasizes its importance in extending, and even saving, lives. Certainly counseling has improved the quality of these women's lives.

All the mothers mentioned emotional benefits of being comforted leading to less worry and more peace. Counseling helped them make choices and prepare for "a new life." They gained information about good diet, disclosure, sex, condoms, and caring for themselves. They believed counseling helped them to become healthier and stronger and to increase their immunity. The counseling has given them access to other beneficial services, such as medical treatment and the support group for PLHA.

Choosing Children or Not. Naomi is a 34-year-old widow with three children aged 14, 12, and 6. Her last-born is HIV-positive, and she believes that because of his sudden death, another child who died at age 6 months was HIV-infected. She lives with the double burden of living with her own HIV and caring for her HIV-infected daughter. Naomi became worried that she might be HIV-infected when she overheard people at her husband's funeral suggesting that her husband had AIDS. His doctor confirmed this to her and asked her to forgive her husband. Naomi recommended that it is better for the mother and father to be tested together.

> *"If the person lives with a husband in marriage, it is best for both to think about their health. They need to be open, to love each other and take care of their children. I would have liked this because if I had known I was HIV positive I wouldn't have planned to get another child."*

Knowledge within couples of their HIV status facilitates discussion, decision making, and caring within the family. This is expected to lead to a longer life and a better quality of life.

In Martina's case, decisions about having children are not only the domain of the wife and husband. The whole family may be involved, applying pressure to have a child.

> *"His family fought with us, saying, 'We need a grandchild.'"*

When asked how many children Martina had planned to have, she was shocked to be asked. She did not perceive herself as being allowed or included in such decisions.

> *"Me? You want to know what I wanted ... (pause) ... With our custom, it's not easy. The husband and relatives decide. The mother doesn't plan a limit. She isn't given an opportunity to say ... I, if I was blessed, I would have liked 2 children—a boy and a girl. Me, myself."*

The context of the research interview allows her the space to consider what her own desires were before she knew her HIV status. She appeared to accept that her reproductive choices were outside of her control and would not even be considered in her marriage or extended family. It is likely the custom she refers to is primarily Islamic, as Tanzanians of other religious backgrounds withstand less pressure and control in reproductive matters.

All the women interviewed demonstrated knowledge that there could be HIV transmission at the time of childbirth; five knew transmission could occur during breastfeeding and four during pregnancy. All understood that there is medicine that can lengthen adult lives and prevent HIV transmission to children. None of the women knew the names or regimens of these medicines but showed intense interest in learning how they work and are used, their benefits and side-effects. Some were aware of women who were included in a pilot study at a hospital in Dar es Salaam. These women used antiretroviral drugs for a few months when pregnant and then gave their child formula milk.

All but one of the women showed concern about the adverse effect of pregnancy on HIV-positive women, particularly if she has AIDS.

> *"For a woman with AIDS to get pregnant is to seek death. Her immunity will drop a lot. For a mother with just the virus it won't be a problem yet, so she can bear a child and continue on. When I was pregnant, I didn't have any health problems. Just the usual." (Sofi)*

> *"It (the pregnancy) can contribute to getting sicker much quicker. If I were planning a child, it would not be good to reduce my immunity, especially in the 6th month." (Martina)*

The belief that pregnancy can hasten illness and death for women with HIV or AIDS is a deterrent to becoming pregnant. Sofi indicates that she believes that she was infected with HIV while pregnant but that this didn't affect her health. She reasons, therefore, that pregnancy is dangerous for women who are already ill with advanced AIDS symptoms.

The reality of sickness has affected the women's previous and future plans for children

> *"Before the sickness (of my husband) we planned to have three children because of the cost of education. When our third child died, it was natural to add another one to get three children. Now after testing, I have no plan to get another child. I guess I don't want more children. I want the ones I have to have the capacity to live so we continue to live this way." (Naomi)*

> *"My view was to advise him to have three children. There was a change of plans after the children died. This change was after the health problems of my husband. We didn't think about having a child. It was because of his health." (Sofi)*

For both Sofi and Naomi, prior to knowing their own HIV status, when one of their children died, they became pregnant again. Sofi's two children died as babies, and she believes they were HIV-infected.

The deaths of these children didn't lead their mothers to consider an underlying possibility of HIV. Rather, these mothers sought to continue to pursue their goal for a certain number of children. Only the illness or deaths of their husbands changed their intentions to have further children.

> *"When my husband married me, he had a wife who had TB and after a short time she died. I was very young ... I remember when I was pregnant; my sister-in-law said, 'Let's see if this child lives.' ... My first child was born safely. He had good health at the beginning. My health was as usual. Then my child was getting disturbing health problems ... We saw he had meningitis ... then he died. My second child had good health ... Just fat! She died in hospital at 9 pm at night. She died while I held her. Both were 4 months ... but without me having any problem with my health..."*

Sofi married at a very young age to be the second wife to a Muslim man. Tuberculosis is taken as a sign that the first wife was HIV-infected. Apparently, other family members wondered whether she, and her children, were infected with HIV. This relates to a belief that living children are a sign that their parents are HIV-free. The contrary belief is that when a child dies, HIV infection may be considered as the cause. The belief that a healthy child is a sign that the HIV virus is not in the family was acknowledged as a common belief within the feedback and focus group. This belief is also evident with both Karol and Madala, who think that their previous partners might be HIV-negative because these men are not sick and both have remarried and have healthy children. During both pregnancies and childbirths, Sofi enjoyed good health, which she seems to find surprising considering the quick decline and early deaths of her children.

Sofi has mixed feelings about having another child. She weighs her desire and ability to have children against the consequences.

> *"If medicine was available, I have a strong desire to get a child ... if it would be possible to get another child, so that my name could continue, but a child could be infected and I would need to have the ability to look after my child. Like ... it is possible that I will perhaps live for 3 years or 2 or 1 year. I can't do this. If I bear a child I will give them suffering in their body—it's not the same as another person."*

Sofi recognizes that issues of reproduction are different for a person with HIV, such as she. She expresses her desire for another child in reference to her future death. She does not have a child to carry on her lineage, as all of her children have died. She again refers to her future anticipated death as an argument against having further children because of concern that she will not be present to care for any children, whether they would be infected or not.

Martina and Karol have already experienced difficulties caring for their children during periods of sickness. To resolve this, Martina's 15-year-old child has lived with his grandmother and now is with an aunt. Karol's older child was taken away by his father, and she attributes this to her sickness at the time.

> *"He took the child when he was 7 years old, after knowing my health was bad. He didn't have a child in his marriage. I had to agree. It wasn't easy to give him up. I gave him up with tears. My mother was very angry. What else could I do when I was so sick?" (Karol)*

The advice the women give on the basis of their own experience is for couples (or the woman) to be tested before becoming pregnant. This gives an opportunity to make informed choices about sexual behavior and childbearing and be able to look after each other. The women did not suggest testing as a basis for choosing medical intervention during pregnancy, which is rarely available as yet. Sofi, however, clearly describes the dilemma about this advice

> *"In marriages people depend on what? The benefits of children. I don't think they would agree." (Sofi)*

When people are well they may not perceive themselves as at risk of having HIV. At a time when couples are planning to begin a new life, they are unlikely to think of the possibility of transmitting a disease that is instead associated with death.

DISCUSSION

Behavior Changes are Needed

Faithfulness to a husband or partner is no guarantee of protection from HIV infection. Five of the women interviewed stated that they made no change in sexual behavior once they found out their HIV status. They had been doing what AIDS prevention messages advise them to do—to be faithful to one partner—but this had not protected them from HIV infection. Married women are a vulnerable population, vulnerable to the effects of their partners' behavior. The Tanzanian Reproductive and Child Health Survey (1999) found that the main reason women felt a moderate or great risk of having HIV was that their partners had other partners, whereas men's perceived risk was related to their own behavior, of having unprotected sex with more than one partner (NBS, 1999). There is a danger in relying on presumptions of monogamy in AIDS prevention messages. "Insist on safer sex" may be a more appropriate message than "Be faithful." However, even insistence on safer sex proved difficult for Martina, who found that her partner refused to use condoms at her request. The difficulty that women have in insisting on safe sex only further strengthens the study participants' recommendations on the need for couple testing and counseling.

The belief that a healthy child is a sign that both the mother and father are HIV-negative was commonly held among the study participants. The belief that a healthy child signifies HIV-negative status in the father could be related to another common belief that the HIV virus is extremely contagious, between men and women and to their children. Slang terms for HIV illustrate this understanding that HIV spreads as fast and sure as "electricity," "wire." or "TANESCO" (the Electricity Commission). Such a belief can delay adults from perceiving that they may already be infected with HIV if they or their children are well. It functions as false reassurance of an HIV-free status and denial that they could be infected. Such cultural beliefs highlight the need for widespread community education on the basic facts about HIV transmission and prevention so that people will not be further constrained from perceiving the risks of HIV infection in their own lives or be immobilized to take action to reduce their own risk or the risk to others.

Changes in Family Planning Intentions. For the mothers in this study, knowledge of their positive HIV status changed or confirmed their intentions not to have further children, while not always changing their desires to have children. For some of the women in this study, the illness or death of their husbands had already affected their initial plans about the size of their family.

A study in West Africa, in Cote d'Ivoire, found that the knowledge of HIV status changed women's desires, relationships, and intentions to have further children. (Aka-Dago-Akribi, Du Lou, Msellati,

Dossou, & Welfens-Ekra, 1999). Another study in West Africa, in Burkina Faso, followed up 306 HIV-positive women after childbirth (Nebie, et al., 2001). This found that during the three-year study, their pregnancy incidence remained comparable to that of the general population. The only factors that prevented pregnancy were severe immunodeficiency and change in marital status.

Prior to knowing their own HIV status, several mothers in this study did not consider the possibility of HIV infection when their own children had died. Instead, their children's deaths only encouraged them to have further children. When there are societal demands for high fertility and for women to fulfill the role of motherhood, a child's death will obviously lead to the need for a replacement. The study in Burkina Faso previously mentioned found that even when women knew their positive HIV status, a poor outcome of a previous pregnancy (such as miscarriage or infant death) was a predictor for another pregnancy.

For the women with only one or no living children, the desire to have children was still strong, which is unsurprising in a society where fertility is highly valued and motherhood is a sign of adulthood. What counteracted this desire or changed women's intentions in family planning were concerns both for themselves and any future children. The women's concerns for themselves included the belief that pregnancy could affect their own health and the difficulties of caring for a baby when they already had other children who needed care. Concerns for future children were the possibility they could be infected with HIV and or be left as orphans if their mothers have only a limited time left to live.

Testing of Couples. The HIV-positive women interviewed recommend concurrent partner testing and disclosure. The testing of women alone has a limited effect, particularly for making plans and decisions and changing behaviour. Testing and knowing HIV serostatus by one partner may not be enough to influence behavior change (Kyaddondo, Rwabukwali, Achom, & Nakabiito, 2000), especially the use of condoms. A Cote d'Ivoire study highlighted that monogamous women are at risk owing to their partners' behavior. This indicates the need to address the couple as a unit, to reduce transmission of HIV to children (Diaby, Painter, Sibailly, et al., 2000) as well as transmission to women. The HIV-positive women in this study recommend greater involvement of men in testing. Present education and communication efforts need to consider how to target testing for couples.

The HIV-positive women desired open and free communication with their partners about sexual and family matters and HIV status. They recommend this communication for others and believe counseling and testing as couples facilitate such communication. Open communication about sexual matters is not a usual part of relationships in Tanzania. The women are suggesting a modification of the norms and context surrounding individual behavior and choices. Women are not alone in this desire. Authors of a study in Harare, Zimbabwe, reported in Durban that male factory workers felt VCT should be offered to couples to help solve communication problems. They wanted HIV test results to assist them plan their family's future (Machekano, McFarland, Bassett, & Mandel, 2000).

At what stage should VCT be targeted and offered to couples? Learning from their own experiences, the mothers in this study recommended that couples be tested for HIV prior to having children. They recognized however, that many would not see the need to do this, especially when healthy. Even so, the earlier that VCT is accepted and accessed, the more benefit can be gained to prevent transmission and to change behavior. Piot of WHO stated, "The single most cost-effective thing that can be done to prevent mother-to-child transmission of HIV is to stop parents becoming infected" (Piot & Coll-Seck, 1999). For the community, there is maximum benefit in primary prevention of HIV in adults, followed by avoiding pregnancy (if HIV-positive), then facilitating medical intervention in pregnancy and counseling about infant feeding and re-infection after delivery. HIV testing and counseling is crucial at every stage: before sexual contact in relationships, before marriage, before pregnancy, during pregnancy, and after delivery. VCT should specifically include counseling about communication and behavior of individuals and couples, whether test results show they are HIV-positive or -negative. Counseling could also address reproductive behavior and choices.

VCT and Access to Services

The mothers in the study outline many benefits to themselves and their families in knowing their HIV status. The timing of their HIV tests meant this knowledge was too late to prevent HIV transmission to their children, even had suitable services been available. However just as important, knowing their own HIV status has enabled these women to access services to extend their lives and improve the quality of their lives and that of their children. It has also apparently influenced them to decide not to have any more children at this stage. VCT is the entry point to accessing a variety of services.

UNICEF is recommending HIV testing and counseling as part of routine hospital antenatal care services (UNICEF, 1999). Hospitals have some existing capacity for VCT and are situated in urban areas where HIV prevalence rates are generally higher (UNICEF, 1999). The precipitating factors that led most of the women in this study to get HIV testing was their own illness or that of their partners. This probably means their testing was occurring when HIV infection may already have been well established. Routine testing would be likely to diagnose women at much earlier stages of infection. The opportunity to counsel and test pregnant women for HIV is not only an opportunity to provide access to prevention strategies such as antiretroviral drugs and infant feeding options. There is also the potential to provide family planning advice, to encourage all women and couples to practice safer sex to prevent new infections or increased viral load, and to provide appropriate clinical care for HIV-positive mothers.

A study in Zimbabwe is exploring the role antenatal care services can play in fostering couple communication and HIV prevention behaviours (Population Council, 2001). Research conducted with pregnant women, men, community leaders and antenatal care staff show that there is widespread interest in increasing male involvement but real challenges exist. Pregnancy and childbirth are perceived as women's domain, with consequent concern by men about loss of respect by being involved in "women's issues" (Population Council). Discussion with partners about safer sex is prohibitive because it implies lack of trust. In a study in Dar es Salaam, most VCT clients interviewed indicated they found it difficult to discuss HIV testing with partners without threatening the relationship. The major concern was fear of the partner's reaction. Women fear abuse or abandonment. Men fear that their partners will panic. Although there is considerable fear of a partner's reaction, the study showed there is little evidence that disclosure frequently leads to physical violence (Maman, Mbwambo, Hogan et al., 2001).

The high levels of HIV prevalence among women of childbearing age in many parts of the world have been described as a triple tragedy (Stover et al., 2003). Not only do women bear the consequences of being HIV-infected, such as stigma, illness, and the prospect of early death. They also may pass the HIV infection on to their children or leave them as orphans. The four-pronged strategy approach of the

United Nations agencies to prevent transmission of HIV to children acknowledges the wisdom in viewing mothers and children as a unit and to therefore take a wide approach to prevention that includes care. The 2001 UN Declaration of Commitment on HIV/AIDS recognized that reducing mother-to-child HIV transmission requires increasing women's access to antenatal care, information, counseling and testing, other prevention services and treatment (UNAIDS, 2001).

The issues involved in HIV prevention, testing, and counseling; drug therapy; provision of services; family planning; and men's participation are a complex web of issues, risks, and benefits. Antiretroviral drugs can be part of a package of care and education with numerous beneficial results beyond reducing HIV transmission to children. There would be maximum effect where access to antenatal care and family planning services are also integrated with HIV testing and counseling facilities. In light of the suggestions made by the interviewed HIV-positive women, we recommend studies examine the comparative advantage of VCT for couples as against VCT for only one partner. Further studies could address the issues involved in achieving more involvement from men in antenatal care and family planning services and increasing access and use of VCT.

CONCLUSION

Arising from their own experiences, these HIV-positive women suggest that counseling and HIV testing offered as a component of programs to prevent mother-to-child HIV transmission would provide additional benefits, especially to the pregnant woman and her partner, beyond reducing HIV transmission to her unborn child. Counseling and HIV testing of couples is considered preferable in order to encourage open communication and to make plans and informed choices together concerning sexual behavior and childbearing. Men's participation in prevention of HIV transmission is considered crucial to facilitate discussion and informed decision making, which can encourage open use of interventions and behavior changes. Complex issues surround future introduction of antiretroviral drugs and other interventions to prevent HIV transmission to children and the expansion and integration of VCT services with family planning and antenatal care services. The issues of integration of services needs to be explored and understood further. This will maximize their acceptability and appropriate use and provide women (and their partners) with greater opportunity for informed choices.

REFERENCES

Aka-Dago-Akridi, H., Du Lou, A., Msellati, P., Dossou, R., et al. (1999). Issues surrounding reproductive choice for women living with HIV in Abidjan, Cote d'Ivoire. *Reproductive Health Matters, 7*(13), 20–29.

Awusabo-Asare, K., & Anarfi, J. (1999). Routes to HIV transmission and intervention: An analytical framework. In I. Orubuloye, J. Caldwell, & J. Ntozi (Eds.), *The continuing HIV/AIDS epidemic in Africa: Responses and coping strategies* (pp. 1–8). Canberra: Health Transition Centre, Australian National University.

Diaby, K., Painter, T., Sibailly, T., et al. (2000). Obstacles to preventing mother-to-child transmission of HIV-1 (MTCT): HIV risk and prevention among pregnant women at a mother-child clinic in Abidjan, Cote D'Ivoire. Abstract No. ThPeC5331 from *Abstracts, Vol. 2, XIII International AIDS Conference*, Durban, July 9–14, 2000.

Guay, L., Musoka, P., Fleming, T., et al. (1999). Intrapartum and neonatal single-dose Nevirapine compared with zidovudine for prevention of mother-to-child transmission of HIV-1 in Kampala, Uganda: HIVNET 012 randomised trial. *The Lancet, 354*(9181), September 4, 1999: 795–802.

Kyaddondo, D., Rwabukwali, C., Achom, M., & Nakabiito, C. (2000). To tell or not to tell? Abstract No. MoPeD2524 from *Abstracts, Vol. 2, XIII International AIDS Conference*, Durban, July 9–14, 2000.

Machekano, R., McFarland, W., Bassett, M., & Mandel, J. (2000). Views and attitudes towards HIV voluntary counselling and testing among urban men: Harare, Zimbabwe. Abstract No. TuPeD3768 from *Abstracts, Vol. 2, XIII International AIDS Conference*, Durban, July 9–14, 2000.

Maman, S., Mbwambo, J., Hogan, M., et al. (2001). HIV and partner violence: Implications for HIV voluntary counseling and testing programs in Dar es Salaam, Tanzania. Washington, D.C.: The Population Council, Inc.

Mandelbrot, L., Le Chenadec, J., Berrebi, A., et al. (1998). Perinatal HIV-1 transmission: Interaction between zidovudine prophylaxis and mode of delivery in the French perinatal cohort. *JAMA, 280*, 55–60.

Marseille, E., Kahn, J., Mmiro, F., et al. (1999). Cost effectiveness of single-dose Nevirapine regimen for mothers and babies to decrease vertical HIV-1 transmission in sub-Saharan Africa. *The Lancet, 354*(9181), 803–809.

National Bureau of Statistics (Tanzania) and Macro International Inc. (1999). *Tanzania Reproductive and Child Health Survey*. Calverton, MD: National Bureau of Statistics (Tanzania) and Macro International Inc.

Nebie, Y., Meda, N., Leroy, V., Mandlebrot, L., et al. (2001). Sexual and reproductive life of women informed of their HIV seropositivity: A prospective cohort study in Burkina Faso. *Journal of Acquired Immune Deficiency Syndrome 28*, 367–372.

Oakley, A. (1981). Interviewing women: A contradiction in terms, In H. Roberts (Ed.), *Doing Feminist Research*. Routledge, London; 30–61.

Piot, P., & Coll-Seck, A. (1999). Preventing Mother-to-child Transmission of HIV in Africa. *Bulletin of the W.H.O., 77*(11), 869.

Population Council. (2001). *Horizons Report Spring 2001*, Washington, DC: The Population Council Inc.

Stover, J., Fuchs, N., Halperin, D., et al. (2003). *Costs and benefits of providing family planning services* at PMTCT and VCT sites. USAID, Office of HIV-AIDS Issues Brief, 2003.

UNAIDS (Joint United Nations Programme on HIV/AIDS). (2000). *Report on the Global HIV/AIDS Epidemic.* June, 2000. Geneva: Author.

UNAIDS (Joint United Nations Programme on HIV/AIDS). (2000). *The International Partnership against AIDS in Africa Update.* Geneva: Author.

UNAIDS (Joint United Nations Programme on HIV/AIDS). (2001). *Declaration of Commitment on HIV/AIDS.* United Nations General Assembly Special Session on HIV/AIDS, June 25–27. Geneva: Author.

UNAIDS (Joint United Nations Programme on HIV/AIDS). (2004). *2004 Report on the global AIDS epidemic.* Geneva: Author.

UNAIDS (Joint United Nations Programme on HIV/AIDS). (2006). 2006 Report on the global AIDS epidemic: A UNAIDS 10th anniversary special edition. Geneva: Author.

UNICEF (United Nations Children's Fund). (1999). *Prevention of mother to child transmission of HIV through breastfeeding.* Dar es Salaam: Author.

Wadsworth, Y. (1997). *Everyday evaluation on the run.* Melbourne: Action Research Issues Association.

Water Aid. (2000). *Tanzania looking back.* London: Water Aid.

Analysis of HIV Caregivers in South Africa: A South African Depression and Anxiety Group

Lisa M. Webb-Robins
Zane Wilson

There is little debate regarding the severity of the HIV/AIDS epidemic in South Africa. The latest data from Statistics South Africa detail a significant feature in the epidemic-its rapid evolution. Recent reports indicate that a national adult HIV prevalence of less than 1% in 1990 increase rapidly to almost 25% within 10 years. A recent study of death registration data found that deaths among people 15 years of age and older increased by 62% in 1997–2002, with deaths among people aged 25–44 years more than doubling. Based on information from nearly 2.9 million death notification certificates, the study showed that more than one third of all deaths were among people in that age group (Statistics SA, 2005). The impact on women is particularly profound. In a recent report produced by the UN Population Fund indicated that nearly 60% of present HIV/AIDS infections are present in women, and most of them are younger (UN, 2005). In southern Africa, young women between the ages of 15 and 24 are at least three times more likely to be HIV-positive than men of the same age.

South Africa faces enormous challenges in scaling up its response to the HIV/AIDS epidemic. Effective responses to HIV/AIDS in low- and middle-income countries have been greatly undermined by specific weaknesses in the area of human resources in medical professions. The South African government has taken several measures to combat this trend, including introducing rural and scarce skills allowances designed to attract and retain health professionals in the public health sector (WHO, 2005). Despite these measures, the country continues to lose skilled health care professionals to wealthier countries, leaving severe shortages in an already overburdened public health system. The WHO also indicates that the current distribution of health workers is heavily weighted in a few urban areas, limiting coverage and "making the integration of treatment with prevention more difficult." Their proposal is to shift to a "standardized and integrated approach to service delivery" that would involve the better use of the human resources that exist, including the simplification of treatment regimens that would rely upon an "expanded clinical team including nursing staff, community members as well as people living with HIV/AIDS employed and trained to perform community outreach and treatment support" (WHO). Despite this positive step in vocalizing the need for utilization of community members, most responses to the proposed effort have been greatly under-resourced and lacking in implementation.

The use of community response through lay caregivers is a key element to mobilization of present resources. While the bulk of the literature on the HIV/AIDS pandemic and support continues to be largely focused on the patients themselves, there have been a number of studies that have sought to uncover the characteristics of caregivers (Flemengas, 2004; SABC News, 2005; Katapa, 2004). Research indicates that most caregivers are women in their childbearing years, which has been found to be the age group most significantly affected by the disease in South Africa (UNAIDS, 2005). Reports evaluating the role of HIV/AIDS caregivers in Africa and other developing world regions have demonstrated that caring for those with AIDS is a substantial burden (Chimwaza and Watkins, 2004; Lindsey, Hirschfeld, & Tlou, 2003; Katapa) with significant impacts upon family and friends of those who have accepted the role. However, other surveys of the literature indicate that the majority of the studies report that caregivers report a sense of pride in their role despite conditions of poverty, social isolation, stigma, and psychological distress (Biel-Cunningham, 2003).

This study seeks to evaluate characteristics, similarities, and differences between the groups of caregivers in rural Kwa Mhlanga (Mpumulanga province), semi-rural Witbank (Mpumulanga province), and urban Johannesburg (Gauteng province) areas of South Africa.

The South African Depression and Anxiety Group (SADAG) has been in existence since 1994 with the main mission to promote mental health through effective country-wide advocacy (http://www.anxiety. org.za/about.profile.php#). SADAG's goals are achieved through a nationwide network of more than 100 patient-led support groups, 40 of which are rural outreach groups in some of South Africa's remotest areas. A key area of concern for SADAG is the overlap between HIV/AIDS, depression, and suicide. In order to address this area of need, SADAG has begun education programs in communities across South Africa with significant focus on home-based HIV/AIDS lay caregivers. Since 1997. SADAG has initiated rural development projects in communities where there are little or no mental health care services available. These programs have been recognized and endorsed by the World Federation for Mental Health (WFMH) and the World Health Organization (WHO). It is through these relationships that the subject pool was mobilized for this study.

METHOD

Site and Participants

Participants for this study comprised 71 total HIV/AIDS caregivers, of whom 48 were considered rural participants. Two surveys were eliminated owing to incomplete information given by respondent to leave 46 total rural participants. Of these participants, 35 were women

(72.9%) and 11 were men (22.9%). Eleven semi-rural participants (72.7%: n = 8 women; 27.3%: n = 3 men) and 14 urban participants (57.1%: n = 8 women; 42.9%: n = 6 men) meeting inclusion criteria participated, and all survey forms were completed. Each participant was an active caregiver to one or more HIV-positive individuals in the community. Inclusion criteria were active caregiver (per self-report), age 18–70 years, and willingness to provide informed consent. The choice of participants can be considered a random self-selection as everyone was given an opportunity within the areas contacted to participate in the study who met the inclusion criteria.

In KwaMhlanga and Witbank, participants came to a local community center where they were individually interviewed by one of the research team (Webb-Robins, Flemengas, Meehan) in private rooms available in the center. In Johannesburg, interviews were completed by local staff members of the community center owing to center policy restrictions. Community centers are considered safe places where individuals congregate and community meetings are held.

Procedure

Participants in this study were self-selected. One week before the researchers were to arrive in each area, the Traditional Healer or primary support group facilitator in the area with whom the SADAG often has direct contact was phoned, and an appointment time was established where community member caregivers were to meet at the community center. A follow-up call the day before was also given to serve as a reminder of the meeting.

Caregivers were individually and privately interviewed by researchers trained in the use of the one-page survey instrument and reflective listening. Depending on the language preference of the participants the survey interview was conducted in either English or Zulu.

Measures

Demographic and Health Characteristics. Demographic information comprised age, gender, occupation and/or employment status, education level, and HIV status using CDC parameters (Centers for Disease Control and Prevention [CDCP], 1998). If caregiver responded in the affirmative to positive HIV status, an additional question regarding date of diagnosis and the health provider and/or Traditional Healer who made the diagnosis was asked.

Living Status. This 10-item scale was extracted from the SADAG Community Questionnaire for Professionals to assess the present physical living situation of the respondent including queries about the presence of electricity, water, toilet, employment, and house construction (e.g. tin, clay, brick). The SADAG measure has effectively been used in the screening of several hundred caregivers and has effectively been utilized as a general measure of present living conditions.

Substance Use History. Select questions from the "Drug and Alcohol Abuse" section, part B, from the Substance Abuse and Mental Health Center for Substance Abuse Treatment (SAMHSA) Government Performance Response Act (GPRA) was used for assessment of present substance use in the respondent as well as typical amounts consumed per week. SAMHSA evaluation criteria were developed to ascertain the needs of communities that have serious emerging drug problems. While the GPRA has not been validated, it uses many items found in the Addiction Severity Index that has established reliability and validity in diverse populations (McLellan, Luborsky, Cacciola, & Griffith, 1985; Leonhard, Mulvey, Gastfriend, & Shwartz, 2000).

Stressful Life Events. This five-item stressful life events scale was developed for the study measures of the presence or absence of negative life events, such as history of physical abuse or rape by intimate partner, childhood rape, or past suicidal ideation. Of note, none of the participants reported presently feeling suicidal at the time this study data was collected.

Data Analysis

The primary measures of interest in this study were the presence or absence of substance use and significant life events in HIV/AIDS lay caregivers across different regions in South Africa. Independent variables were derived from (1) sociodemographic characteristics (gender, age, years of education, relative poverty indicators); (2) stressful life events; and (3) the presence of substance use. Group comparisons for participants in each area of consideration (rural, semi-rural, and urban) were undertaken using chi-square tests for categorical variables with analysis of each independent variable associated with those three locations. Multivariate analysis (discriminate function analysis) was used to investigate factors found significant that differentiated between groups. Statistical significance was set at the level of $p = 05$ (two-tailed). Data were computed using SPSS version 11.5 for Windows.

RESULTS

Demographic Status

In the rural group, there are significantly more women respondents (72.9%: n = 35) than male respondents (22.9%: n = 11). There were no significant differences between age, living status, or home composition. While there were no findings of statistical significance between areas of house composition and living status, the findings are telling regarding the relative poverty of the individuals surveyed. One item of note is possible difference in perception of the role of caregivers across areas. In rural areas, it appears that most caregivers categorize their caregiving role as their "employment," though most do not realize any financial gain for their services. In contrast, caregivers in semi-rural and urban areas categorize themselves as "unemployed" rather than using their status as a "caregiver" as employment. Regarding HIV status, as the diagnosis is stigmatized it is possible that there was underreporting of positive status, particularly in rural and semi-rural areas. The total percentage of individuals reporting "don't know" to their HIV status in rural and semi-rural areas is also particularly notable. It was evident that there was fear in having knowledge surrounding HIV status and the accompanying stigma associated with a positive diagnosis.

Demographic Characteristics

Reported Life Events. While findings proved to not be significant regarding reported abuse, qualitative questions described patterns of repeated ongoing physical and emotional abuse occurring within the context of their intimate spouse-partner relationship. These patterns ranged from daily to monthly with a number of endorsements for ongoing emotional abuse.

When evaluating comparisons across groups (rural, semi-rural, and urban) regarding ever having thoughts of suicide, there is no significant difference ($p = .102$). However, when evaluating the total number of respondents without categorization into geographic region (rural, semi-rural, and urban), we find that there is a statistical difference between those who have been hurt/not hurt by partner/spouse and those who have had thoughts of suicide in the past ($p = .002$). The measure of correlation (phi value) is .412 (significance of .001). The test of difference remains significant for those respondents in a rural

TABLE 1. Demographic and Diagnostic Characteristics of Caregivers

Variable	Rural (n = 46)	Semi-rural (n = 11)	Urban (n = 14)
Mean age	30.88 years	38.6 years	29.78 years
Mean years education completed	10th grade (range 5th grade–12th grade)	5th grade (range 3rd grade–8th grade, 3 = no education)	9th grade (range 4th grade–college)
Gender (%)			
Male	22.9% (n = 11)	27.3% (n = 3)	42.9% (n = 6)
Female	72.9% (n = 35)	72.7% (n = 8)	57.1% (n = 8)
% unemployment	16.7% (n = 8)	90.9% (n = 10)	92.9% (n = 13)
Caregiver reported as primary employment (%)	72.9% (n = 35)	n/a	7.1% (n = 1)
Living status			
Electricity in home	75% (n = 36)	45.5% (n = 5)	64.3% (n = 9)
Water in home	35.4% (n = 17)	54.5% (n = 6)	57.1% (n = 8)
Toilet in home	20.8% (n = 10)	27.3% (n = 3)	42.9% (n = 6)
Home composition			
House: Brick	62.5% (n = 30)	27.3% (n = 3)	78.6% (n = 11)
House: Clay	8.3% (n = 4)	—	—
House: Tin	10.4% (n = 5)	63.6% (n = 7)	14.3% (n = 3)
House: Soil	6.3% (n = 3)	—	—
House: Clay	2.1% (n = 1)	—	—
House: Other	—	9.1% (n = 1)	7.1% (n = 1)
HIV status			
% reporting positive	8.3%	36%	100%
% reporting negative	59.5%	18%	0%
% unknown status	31%	45%	0%

location only (*p* value of .020). Furthermore, the variables remain correlated (phi value of .427; *p* value of .005). There are no statistical differences for those respondents in a semi-rural environment (*p* value of .406) or for those who live in an urban location.

When evaluating the total number of respondents without categorization into geographic region (rural, semi-rural, and urban), we find that there is also a statistical difference between those who have been raped and have not and thoughts of suicide (*p* value = .035). The variables are also correlated, with a Phi value of .296 and a *p* value of .014. If, however, we select only those in the rural location, there is no significant difference between those who have/have not been raped and thoughts of suicide and the variables are not correlated (*p* value of .170) nor for semi-rural (*p* value of 1.00) or for urban (*p* value of 1.0).

On qualitative explanations regarding why caregivers have felt suicidal in the past, primary responses surrounded issues of stigmatization for HIV diagnosis, unemployment/lack of financial resources, despair due to the loss of loved ones to HIV, and a general loss of hope. It is important to note, however, that though there was a positive endorsement of previous thoughts of suicide in the caregivers surveyed, when asked if there were present thoughts of suicide respondent responded in the negative with a "no" response.

Substance Use Factors. When evaluating the differences between rural, semi-rural, and urban caregivers and their alcohol use, Tests for Differences procedures were completed in SPSS to select only the relevant caregivers and *t*-tests for two Independent Sample Means ("Location of your Town" variable = nominal level; "How Many Times a Week Do You Drink Alcohol" = ratio level). On average, it appears that semi-rural caregivers drink alcohol more times a week than rural (3.25 compared to 1.1667), significant at the .05 level. However, there was no qualifier in the survey indicating "how much" alcohol was consumed in each "time per week," thus potentially underestimating the amount actually consumed. Comparing rural to urban and semi-rural to urban alcohol use was also not found to be significant (.314, .074, respectively). Evaluating marijuana use yielded a result that was also not found to be significant, probably in part owing to small cell counts in some of the cells. No caregivers reported using cocaine, and many asked what the drug was, as many had never heard of the substance.

TABLE 2. Life Events

Variable	Rural (n = 46)	Semi-rural (n = 11)	Urban (n = 14)
Abuse, (physical and emotional) (%)	12.5%	27.3%	14.3%
Spouse/partner rape (%)	27.1%	18.2%	28.6%
Rape as child (%)	8.3%	9.1%	7.1%
Ever had thoughts of suicide (%)	37.5%	63.6%	21.4%

TABLE 3. Reported Substance Use in Participant Caregivers

Variable	Rural	Semi-rural	Urban
Alcohol use (%)	20.8% (n = 10)	36.4% (n = 4)	71.4% (n = 11)
Average consumption times per week	3	1	2
Marijuana use (%)	2.1% (n = 1)	18.3% (n = 2)	14.3% (n = 2)
Cocaine use (%)	0%	0%	0%
Sniff glue	0%	27.3% (n = 3)	0%
Sex while intoxicated (%)	4.2% (n = 2)	36.4% (n = 4)	28.6% (n = 4)

DISCUSSION

The primary measures of interest in this study were the presence or absence of significant life events and substance use in HIV/AIDS lay caregivers across different regions in South Africa. Group comparisons for participants in each area of consideration (rural, semi-rural, and urban) were undertaken using chi-square tests for categorical variables with analysis of each independent variable associated with those three locations.

In general, our sample consisted of women ranging in age from 22 to 53 years in the rural area, 22 to 62 years in the semi-rural area, and 20 to 48 years in the urban area, with the majority of women being in their younger childbearing years. Most reported limited education, very high unemployment levels, and sparse living conditions, with many living without water or a toilet inside the home.

While findings were not significant regarding reported abuse, qualitative questions regarding the number of times physical abuse occur within their intimate spouse/partner relationship ranged from daily to monthly, with a number of endorsements for emotional abuse. Therefore, it would appear that though the number of individuals reporting abuse is somewhat small, the perceived severity of the abuse is noteworthy. Further, it is possible that there is under-endorsement of this question for concern that the abusive partner would be contacted. Self-administered questionnaires would likely assist in getting more accurate information on this issue.

When evaluating the total number of respondents without categorization into geographic region (rural, semi-rural, and urban), we find that there is a statistical difference between those who have been hurt/not hurt by partner/spouse and those who have had thoughts of suicide. It was also found that those who have been raped in the past by an intimate partner have had thoughts of suicide. These findings indicate a substantial need for further study in the area of suicidality, suicidal thoughts, and the need for a support network within lay caregivers. This finding supports previous data collected by SADAG (Flemengas, 2004).

Several limitations of this study are worth noting. One key limitation to the data analysis of this study stems from the substantial differences in participant group numbers. Rural participants (n = 46) far exceed those in semi-rural (n = 11) or urban (n = 14) areas. Sample sizes make the ability to generalize these findings to larger populations challenging. However, additional support for findings related to caregivers having suicidal thoughts are supported by other studies conducted by SADAG in the past. Should further studies of this type be conducted, a larger sample size to be able to more adequately compare across groups would be advantageous. The interviewer-administered questionnaire format of this study may prove to underestimate significant life events, substance use, and unsafe sexual practices ("Sex while intoxicated") compared with self rated measures that might be more reliable in eliciting information on sexual behavior (Kelly et al., 1992). In addition, the questionnaire for this study was deliberately short to increase study participation. Therefore, additional questions might increase understanding of how stressful life events may impact caregivers' ability to care for others. Further, questions asked were largely from surveys that had been utilized for American populations which may not have accounted for relative cultural issues present in our sample.

In addition, in one study site (Whitbank), the Traditional Healer was present while some interviews were conducted. Each participant had the opportunity to excuse the Traditional Healer and have a more confidential interview, but each chose not to. It is possible that these interviewees may have answered questions in a manner that introduced bias or possible under-reporting of sensitive issues.

While the analysis of substance use in caregivers was not found to be significant, one can see some general trends revealed in the findings of this study. Based upon those surveyed, it appears that there could be an emerging substance use issue within the rural areas, particularly in the area of alcohol consumption. Though the issue of substance use across the country is emerging as a concern (SA Ministry of Health, 2005), lay caregivers could be particularly vulnerable to this issue owing to possible high stress levels and other psychological factors present in their assistance role. Without support groups or networks of individual to share experiences as caregivers, it is possible that the prevalence of substance use in this population may increase.

Overall, interesting trends were noticed in the areas of suicidality, alcohol abuse, and intimate trauma that are worth exploring in future studies with caregivers. These findings indicate a substantial need for further study in the area of suicidality, suicidal thoughts, denial or a lack of desire to know HIV status and the accompanying diagnostic stigma, and the need for a support network within lay caregivers. Findings support previous data collected by SADAG (Flemengas, 2004).

REFERENCES

Biel-Cunningham, S. (2003). The support needs of caregivers: The body: The complete HIV/AIDS resource. Retrieved June 2, 2008, from http://www.thebody.com/content/art32303.html

Centers for Disease Control and Prevention. (1999). Morbidity and Mortality Weekly Report: *Revised Guidelines for HIV Counseling, Testing, and Referral Technical Expert Panel Review of CDC HIV Counseling, Testing, and Referral Guidelines.* February 18–19, Atlanta, Georgia.

Center for Disease Control and Prevention. (1998). AIDS cases reported to the Centers for Disease Control through December 1998. *HIV/AIDS Surveillance Report, 10*(2), 1–43.

Chimwaza A. F., & Watkins, S. C. (2004). Giving care to people with symptoms of AIDS in rural sub-Saharan Africa. *AIDS Care, 16*(7), 795–807.

Department of Health and Department of Social Development, South Africa. (2003). Appraisal of Home/Community-Based Care projects in South Africa 2002–2003. Pretoria, South Africa: Department of Health and Department of Social Development.

Flemengas, M. (2004). The extent of depression in HIV/AIDS home base caregivers in Limpopo, Mpumalanga, Northern cape, and North West Province. *South African Depression and Anxiety Group Newsletter*, May edition.

Katapa, R. S. (2004). Caretakers of AIDS patients in rural Tanzania. *International Journal of STD AIDS, 15*(10), 673–678.

Kelly, J. A., Murphy, D. A., Bahr, R., Brasfield, T. L., Davis, D. R., Hauth, A. C., et al. (1992). AIDS/HIV risk behavior among the chronic mentally ill. *American Journal of Psychiatry, 150*(6), 972–974.

Leonhard, C., Mulvey, K., Gastfriend, D. R., & Shwartz, M. (2000). The Addiction Severity Index: A field study of internal consistency and validity. *Journal of Substance Abuse Treatment, 18*, 129–135.

Lindsey, E., Hirschfeld, M., & Tlou, S. (2003) Home-based care in Botswana: Experiences of older women and young girls. *Health Care for Women International, 24*(6), 486–501.

McLellan, A. T., Luborsky, L., Cacciola, J., & Griffith, J. E. (1985). New data from the Addiction Severity Index: Reliability and validity in three centers. *The Journal of Nervous and Mental Disease, 173,* 412–423.

SABC news: Minister urges youth to take charge of their lives. Retrieved June 25, 2005, from http://www.sabcnews.com/south_africa/health/0,2172,107188,00.html

Statistics South Africa. (2005). Mortality and causes of death in South Africa, 1997–2003. Pretoria: Author.

UNAIDS/WHO. AIDS Epidemic Update. Retrieved December, 2005, from http://www.unaids.org/epi/2005/doc/report_pdf.asp

WHO summary country profile, 2005. Retrieved June 2, 2008, from http://www.who.int/3by5/support/june2005_zaf.pdf Treating 3 million by 2005: Making it happen, The WHO Strategy (2003) http://www.who.int/3by5/publications/documents/en/3by5StrategyMakingItHappen.pdf

WHO, June 2005. Progress on global access to HIV antiretroviral therapy: An update on 3 by 5. Retrieved June 2, 2008, from http://www.who.int/hiv/pub/progress reports/3by5%20Progress%20Report_E_light.pdf

A Model Program for Increasing Treatment Access for African American Women Who Use Crack Cocaine and Are at Risk of Contracting HIV

Samuel Okpaku
Samuel A. MacMaster
Sheila Dennie
Deon Tolliver

There is a growing racial disparity in HIV/AIDS incidence rates that primarily affects African-American women. Although African-Americans represent only 12.3% of the U.S. population, they disproportionately make up approximately 39% of all AIDS cases (Centers for Disease Control [CDC], 2005). For African-American women, this inequality is significantly increased, as African-Americans represent 72% of all female HIV cases nationally and experience rates at 25 times greater than white women (CDC, 2004). In Tennessee, the gap is further widened as African-Americans embody 16% of Tennessee's population, yet account for 81% of AIDS cases among women. Of greater concern, AIDS rates were *28 times greater* for African-American women as compared to white women and 3.5 times greater than other women of color (Tennessee Department of Health, 2002).

Drug use represents a well-established risk behavior for HIV, primarily as it relates to injection drug use. Other drug users are increasingly at high risk for contracting HIV as the awareness of the relationship of non-injection drug use to HIV risk has grown. Specifically, crack cocaine smokers have been found to be three times more likely to be infected with HIV than non-smokers (Friedman et al., 2003). Use of crack cocaine can contribute to the spread of the epidemic when users trade sex for drugs or money, when they engage in risky sexual behaviors that they might not engage in when not under the influence, or when their use affects access to health care services (Ross et al., 1999; Marx et al., 1991; Cottler et al., 1998). Importantly, substance abuse treatment can be effective in reducing HIV risk among crack cocaine users (Hoffman et al., 1998).

However, before an individual can benefit from substance abuse treatment services, they must first gain access to, and become engaged with, these services. Without said opportunity, many women are unable to overcome barriers to treatment access and engagement, therefore continue to use, contract HIV, and die. Currently, AIDS is the leading cause of death of young (25- to 34-year-old) African-American women in this country (National Center for Health Statistics, 2002).

DISPARITIES IN ACCESS TO SUBSTANCE ABUSE TREATMENT SERVICES

There is also a growing awareness of general racial and gender inconsistencies in access to health care that disproportionately affects African-Americans (Institute of Medicine, 2003). While these disparities are important to the larger community, there appear to be other factors that primarily affect African-American women who use crack cocaine. These women are subject to a unique environmental context with specific individual and environmental stressors that have direct and dramatic effect on health outcomes specifically related to HIV/AIDS.

Only a small percentage (18.2%) of the individuals who identify a need for substance abuse treatment are able to access it, and there is a definitive gender difference in rates of treatment admissions (National Survey on Drug Use and Health [NSDUH], 2004). Although women use illicit drugs less frequently than men (6.4% vs. 10.3% of the population) (NSDUH, 2004), analyses of the Treatment Episode Data Set found that from 1992 to 1998, women represented only about 30% of all admissions. Importantly, women are also more likely than men to designate cocaine as their drug of choice (DASIS, 2001).

Racial discrepancies also exist but are less definitive. African-Americans experience substance dependence and abuse at rates slightly higher but generally comparable to Caucawhites, 9.5% versus 9.3% (NSDUH, 2004). Despite these comparable rates, African-Americans enter treatment at disproportionately higher rates, as African-Americans account for 12% of the population but 24% of treatment admissions (TEDS, 2004). However, the rates for substance abuse treatment admissions for African-Americans steadily declined 15% between 1994 and 1999, while rates for admissions for the total population increased three percent (DASIS, 2002). This statistic is skewed by higher rates of involvement in the criminal justice system, as criminal justice referrals were the most frequent referral source for African-Americans, accounting for 37% of all admissions (DASIS, 2002). Therefore, disparities in treatment access are primarily among African-Americans *not* involved in the criminal justice system.

Barriers to Treatment Access

Barriers to treatment access exist that can be conceptualized as either individually or environmentally based. Individually based barriers to treatment access are often conceptualized in terms of treatment readiness or treatment motivation (Zule, Lam, & Wechsberg, 2003; Joe, Simpson, & Boome, 1998) and include the lack of a desire for treatment, income, insurance status, and cultural or peer norms. Additional environmentally based structural barriers exist that prevent access to treatment, such as a fees waiting list (Wechsberg et al., 2001), despite a willingness to enter treatment (MacMaster and Vail, 2002). For African-American crack cocaine users, documented barriers have included a lack of transportation, childcare needs, and/or the ability to self-pay for services (Wechsberg et al., 2003; MacMaster, 2005).

Issues of race and gender that impact the target population may further impact treatment access. Traditional approaches to substance abuse and HIV prevention and substance abuse treatment may be problematic among African-Americans given unfavorable views of available treatments (Longshore, Hsieh, & Anglin, 1993) and distrust of mainstream social services (Aponte & Barnes, 1995). Further traditional middle-class Euro-American intervention and treatment models may be inconsistent with those of many African-Americans (Cochran and Mays, 1993) at risk as these models assume that people have the necessary resources and do not consider the barriers to prevention and intervention. Africentric models have been posited that provide a framework for preventing HIV and substance use risk and may facilitate treatment access and engagement (Belgrave, Brome, & Hampton, 2000; Belgrave, Reed, Plybon, & Corneille, 2004; Belgrave, Townsend, Cherry, & Cunningham, 1997) Beyond culture based on race and ethnicity, there appear to be both a drug using culture and a culture of substance abuse recovery (Holleran and MacMaster, 2005). Perceptions of this cultural congruence may also influence treatment access and engagement.

Traditional HIV and substance abuse services have not met the needs of many women. Despite the increasing rate of HIV infection among women, interventions aimed at reducing the spread of HIV have not always been tailored to be gender-specific. Historically, most HIV education and prevention programs have focused primarily on gay or bisexual male individuals or injection drug users with a resultant lag in the development and identification of successful programs addressing the needs and concerns of women (Amaro, 1995). Similarly, crack cocaine-using men are also more likely to enter substance abuse treatment than women (Wechsberg et al., 2005), and men are also more likely to seek treatment services (Copeland, 1997).

Program Description

The Treatment Access Project for African American Women is designed to provide a coordinated continuum of services to individuals at risk of contracting HIV/AIDS. This is accomplished by building on the core strengths of three existing programs: The Lloyd C. Elam Mental Health Center of Meharry Medical College, which has been providing substance abuse outreach and treatment services since 1972; Metropolitan Interdenominational Church's First Response Center, an African-American, faith-based case management program for persons living with or at risk for HIV/AIDS; and Street Works, an outreach program with late-night and weekend services that targets substance users at risk for contracting HIV. This community-based collaboration leads to (1) increased access to comprehensive substance abuse treatment through the removal of current barriers and (2) an enhanced culturally relevant treatment program that provides an intensive treatment program designed to improve retention in services by enhancing treatment readiness and motivation for change; it includes specific educational interventions focused on HIV/AIDS and hepatitis C.

Purpose and Goals of the Program

The primary goal of the program is to strengthen the existing collaborative partnership among participating organizations to provide a coordinated continuum of culturally competent HIV risk reduction, substance abuse treatment, and other related services to African-American female substance abusers. Ultimately this strengthened collaboration improves the health and HIV/AIDS risk status of the target population through (1) the removal of barriers that reduce the likelihood of members entering and remaining in substance abuse treatment, (2) reduction of the use of alcohol and other drugs, (3) increased motivation to adopt risk-reduction strategies (both substance abuse and sex-related risks), and (4) increased self-sufficiency and psychosocial functioning, including improved employment stability, improved housing stability, decreased involvement with the criminal justice system, and improved mental health status.

Framework for Interventions

The program model is based upon an enhancement of the strategies developed as part of the extensively evaluated National AIDS Demonstration Research (NADR) program and the NIDA Cooperative Agreement for AIDS Community-Based Outreach Intervention Research Program, both of which are regarded as the best practice models for reaching out of treatment substance users (Needle and Coyle, 1997, 1998). The intervention approach is also rooted in the Trans-theoretical, or "stages-of-change" (SOC) model (Prochaska and DiClemente, 1992), viewing changes in addictive behaviors as a process requiring movement through a series five stages of behavior change. Outreach intervention also represents state of the art practices through the implementation of a protocol that takes into account that not all at-risk individuals will be at the same stage of change with regard to their substance abuse or sexual risk behavior. The content of the street intervention is tailored to the participant's current stage of change. Street outreach implies that most at risk individuals are not in treatment and many will be at the pre-contemplation and early contemplation stages. For these individuals, the key challenge is to create the motivation for change. Initial outreach contacts are structured to employ motivational interviewing strategies.

Outreach is followed by pretreatment services, which are an enhancement to existing treatment services. The design utilizes a motivational interviewing approach (Miller and Rollnick, 1991) to delivering pretreatment services and borrows heavily from the experience of Wechsberg and colleagues (2005) in North Carolina. Motivational interviewing is a directive, client-centered counseling style for achieving behavior change by facilitating exploration and resolution of ambivalence. This is a focused and goal-directed approach. Motivation to change is encouraged but comes from the client. It is not imposed externally.

While preexisting Elam Center substance abuse services provided treatment that addressed specific needs associated with HIV/AIDS, and the cultural and gender needs of African-American women. The following new elements were incorporated into the treatment approach:

• Treatment planning addresses needs specifically related to HIV/AIDS, gender, and culture. Treatment planning is negotiated within the context of an individual counseling session between the client and counselor. The client is empowered in the planning process to determine the specific goals and objectives to pursue, while the client serves as a guide to ensure that HIV/AIDS, gender, and culture issues are adequately addressed.

- A strong case management model is integrated into treatment with close coordination occurring between counselor, case manager, and client. The focus of case management is not solely acquiring basic and supportive services, but also addressing integration of those services through educating providers regarding substance abuse recovery and HIV/AIDS needs. Included in case management is the acquisition of services for pregnant women and women with dependent children, including women who are trying to regain custody of their children. These services include: primary medical care, primary pediatric care (including immunizations), therapeutic interventions for children in custody of women in treatment, and sufficient transportation.
- The traditional abstinence based approach to addiction treatment and recovery is softened, where needed, to allow for gradual reduction in substance use. This is to accommodate HIV-infected substance abusers that are "unable to maintain abrupt and total discontinuation of substance abuse."
- A multidisciplinary team meets weekly to address the client's treatment needs. To ensure that the target population receives special attention, the team consists of the Elam Center Medical Director, the assigned counselor, the Project Coordinator, the Director of Women's Services, the Case Manager, the Women's Services Licensed Practical Nurse, workers from Project COPE and SISTER, and representatives from other agencies providing services through established linkages.

Components of the Program

Outreach Activities. One activity is to target African-American women who use substances, specifically crack cocaine. Meharry Outreach teams (SISTER) target African-American women who live in public housing and are currently using alcohol and/or other drugs or who are in early recovery. Street Works targets sex industry workers, many of whom are also using alcohol and other drugs. From the front end of the continuum (outreach activities), this program addresses access-related obstacles of timing and trust. Outreach efforts can be severely handicapped because many members of the population are simply not out in the community during the agencies' hours of operation. Synergy created between Meharry and Street Works Outreach teams allow for a much-increased probability that the target population is reached, because of the 24-hour 7-day-week capabilities of the collaborative. Each agency has established trust in the community relative to specific locations and general times of day/night. By teaming up, obstacles of timing and trust can be turned into opportunities. Larger numbers are reached through expanded human resources, while the chances of engagement are increased through established and trusting relationships between agencies and community.

Pretreatment Services. Once the client is engaged through outreach efforts, she is recruited to pretreatment services. Collaborative efforts continue to address issues of trust yet also begin to establish a support network for the client both by the providers and the clients themselves. The competency the SISTER Program has developed over the years in the area of building support among African-American female substance abusers is legendary. The fact that the majority of SISTER's staff members are themselves recovering African-American females helps enormously in trust- and support-building efforts. This, coupled with Street Works' reputation as a street-savvy agency (with staff who have been-there-and-done-that), facilitates an environment that engages this population in pretreatment interventions. Proven pretreatment intervention techniques such as brief intervention, pre-screening, and motivational interviewing, combined with street smarts, support-building experience, and trust, will facilitate clients' entry into treatment and improve their prognosis for treatment and recovery. Here the goals of access and retention are addressed simultaneously. Motivation for treatment facilitates hope and the desire to access treatment while planting the seeds needed to become engaged in the treatment process.

Case Management. Once the client decides to enter treatment, a First Response Center case manager is assigned to her. The case manager provides continuity between outreach, pretreatment, and treatment. Case management is based on an alcohol and drug abuse services coordination model and is customized to address the specific needs of African-American women, while simultaneously integrating HIV/AIDS services. The case manager performs a needs assessment and develops a case management plan to facilitate the removal of obstacles to the treatment and recovery process, which is directly linked to the goal of retention.

Substance Abuse Treatment. Women have been transitioned to a number of community substance abuse treatment providers; however, the majority have entered treatment at the Elam Center. To remove obstacles to access for a subset of the target population, pregnant and postpartum women, and their children, the capacity of the Elam Center's Rainbow program was expanded. Some of the most difficult substance abuse treatment services to access include long-term residential services for pregnant and postpartum women. The Rainbow program is the only such program in the middle Tennessee area; thus, it continuously operates with a waiting list. Expanding Rainbow's capacity and designating the expansion to African-American women clearly addresses the goal of treatment access as it pertains to the this subset of the target population.

Characteristics of Participants

Demographics. Over the 2 years of the project, seventy-eight individuals completed an initial interview and provided their own demographic information (Table 1). In line with the focus of the project, all participants were women and reported their race as African-Americans; none of the participants indicated that their ethnicity was Hispanic/ Latino. As a group, the participants were young; almost all (76.9%) of respondents were below the age of 45. Average educational attainment was below the high-school level and averaged 11.19 years. Slightly more than one-fourth (26.9%) of the respondents had received a

TABLE 1. Demographics

Demographic	Categories	N = 78 (%)
Age	18–24	11.5
	25–34	25.6
	35–44	39.7
	45–54	21.8
	55–64	1.3
Gender	Female	100
Ethnicity/racial background	African-American	100
Education (yrs)		11.19
Housing status	Housed	80.8
	Homeless	12.8
	Shelter	3.8
	Institution	2.8

TABLE 2. Characteristics of Drug Use in the Last Thirty Days

Demographic	Categories	N = 78 (%)
Used any of the following substances in the last 30 days	Cocaine	84.6
	Alcohol	69.2
	Marijuana	47.4
	Tylenol 2,3,4	9.0
	Benzodiazepines	7.7
	Codeine	6.4
	Morphine	2.6
	Barbiturates	2.6
	Percocet	1.3
	Hallucinogens	1.3
	Inhalants	1.3
	Methamphetamines	1.3
	Tranquilizers	1.3

high-school diploma; however, an additional proportion (9.0%) reported obtaining a GED. The majority (80.8%) of the respondents were housed, with more than one-third (41%) of these individuals housed in their own apartment or home. Those individuals who were permanently housed but did not live in their own home or apartment primarily (32.1%) lived in someone else's home. Almost all (80%) of respondents had children, and one respondent reported being pregnant but, owing to changes in data collection, these questions were asked only of the ten most recent interviewees. Almost all (92.3%) of the respondents were unemployed.

Reasons for Seeking Services. All of the participants reported that they sought treatment on their own and were not coerced into services by the criminal justice system, an employer, or any other entity. All program participants were referred through the street outreach programs described in the collaboration.

Drug Use Characteristics. In concert with the focus of this project, cocaine (84.6%) was the most frequently reported substance used in the last 30 days prior to accessing services. Nearly one-third of respondents (16.7%) reported using daily. High levels of alcohol (69.2%) and marijuana (47.4%) accounted for almost all of the remaining reported drug use. There was no reported use of heroin, and one individual reported using methamphetamines.

Implications for Practice

All too often when working with individuals, practitioners focus on the immediate social and environmental needs of that person with less emphasis on their needs both short and long term. Clients with complex problems need comprehensive holistic services that help people reassemble their lives; thus, access to substance abuse treatment is truly only the tip of the iceberg. Some individuals are so severely traumatized by poverty, family issues, and arrested psychological, social, and spiritual development that any change requires intensive interventions. Individuals need tremendous, long-term support because of their sense of hopelessness. Immediate services are needed or the transitory motivation to change is lost. Immediate treatment and housing are needed to start the process of change and later, long-term support, resource identification, and acquisition are necessary. Because of these needs, moving people from "hopelessness" to a "hopeful" state requires long-term relationship-based services that contain a spiritual component. Moving an individual through this process of spiritual change is related to behavioral changes that they experience. The movement from hopeless to hopeful is much more than simple access to services; rather it requires a reorganization of that individual's relationship with their environment.

Of significance is the model of services that was developed by the aforementioned project. This project was also able to develop a non-coercive model for providing culturally competent services to chronic African-American female crack cocaine users who have not had their needs met by other service delivery models. The project was able to connect with these individuals, retain them in intensive case management services, transition them to substance abuse services, and provide continual supports as they became productive members of the community. While there has been much discussion about the need for culturally competent and faith-based services targeted for African-American substance users, this project is able to provide data that supports the efficacy of the use of this method.

CONCLUSION

This article has offered a description of the Treatment Access Project, a community-based program providing a comprehensive set of services targeted to a African-American female population of active cocaine users. While previous research has shown that targeted out-reach efforts can be effective, this article provides a description of an array of services designed to be culturally relevant within the African-American community by incorporating a gender-specific approach to service delivery. Active drug users, as a group, are often reluctant to connect with services. The program described in this article provides an example of how services can be provided to individuals in a culturally relevant and non-coercive manner.

REFERENCES

Albelda, R., & Tilly, C. (1997). Glass ceiling and bottomless pits: Women's work, women's poverty. Boston: South End Press.

Aponte, J. F., & Barnes, J. M. (1995). Impact of acculturation and moderator variables on the intervention and treatment of ethnic groups. In J. F. Aponte, R. Y. River, & J. Wohl (eds.), *Psychological Interventions and Cultural Diversity*, 19–39. Boston: Allyn & Bacon.

Belgrave, F. Z., Brome, D., & Hampton, C. (2000). The contributions of Africentric values and racial identity to the prediction of drug knowledge, attitudes and use among African American youth. *Journal of Black Psychology, 26*(4), 386–401.

Belgrave, F. Z., Reed, M. C., Plybon, L. E., & Corneille, M. (2004). The impact of a culturally enhanced drug prevention program on drug and alcohol refusal efficacy among urban African American girls. *Journal Drug Education, 34,* 267–279.

Belgrave, F. Z., Townsend, T. G., Cherry, V. R., & Cunningham, D. M. (1997). The influence of an Africentric world-view and demographic variables on drug knowledge, attitudes, and use among African American youth. *Journal of Community Psychology, 25(5),* 421–433.

Bureau of Justice Statistics. (2004). HIV in Prisons and Jails, 2002.

Bureau of Justice Statistics. (2004). Prisoners in 2003.

Bok, M., & Morales, J. (1997). The Impact and implications of HIV on children and adolescents: Social justice and social change. *Journal of HIV/AIDS Prevention & Education for Adolescents & Children, 1*(1), 9–34.

Bull, C. (2003). An AIDS wake-up call. *Advocate, 885,* 35–37.

Burston, B., Jones, D., & Roberson-Saunders, P. (1995). Drug use and African Americans: Myths and reality. *Journal of Alcohol and Drug Education, 40,* 19–39.

Campbell, C. A. (1999). *Women, families, and HIV/AIDS: A sociological perspective on the epidemic in America.* Cambridge: University Press.

Centers for Disease Control. Health, United States, 2004: Table 30. (2004). Hyattsville, MD: U.S. Department of Health and Human Services, CDC, National Center for Health Statistics. Retrieved from ... http://www.cdc.gov/nchs/data/hus/hus04trend.pdf#03.

Centers for Disease Control. (2004). Health disparities experienced by racial/ethnic minority populations. *Morbidity and Mortality Weekly Report 53*:755.

Centers for Disease Control and Prevention. (2004). CDC HIV/AIDS among African Americans.

Centers for Disease Control and Prevention. (2005). *HIV/AIDS Surveillance Report: 2004, 16*(2).

Centers for Disease Control. (2005). Health disparities experienced by African Americans—United States. *Morbidity and Mortality Weekly Report, 54*:1–3.

Chu, S. Y., & Curran, J. W. (1997). The epidemiology of HIV. In DeVita, Jr., Hellman, and Rosenberg (Eds.), AIDS: Biology, diagnosis, treatment and prevention (4th ed.). Philadelphia: Lippincott-Raven Publishers.

Cochran, S. D., & Mays, V. M. (1993). Applying social psychological models to predicting HIV-related sexual risk behaviors among African-Americans. *Journal of Black Psychology, 19*, 142–154.

Copeland, J. (1997). A qualitative study of barriers to formal treatment among women who self-managed change in addictive behaviors. *Journal of Substance Abuse Treatment, 110*, 445–448.

Cottler, L. B., Leukefeld, C., Hoffman, J., Desmond, D., Wechsberg, W., Inciardi, J., Compton, W. M., Ben Abdallah, A., Cunningham-Williams, R., & Woodson, S. (1998). Effectiveness of HIV risk reduction initiatives among out-of-treatment non-injection drug users. *Journal of Psychoactive Drugs 1998, 30*(3): 279–290.

Diaz, T., Chu, S., Buehler, J., et al. (1994). Socioeconomic differences among people with AIDS: Results from a multistate surveillance project. *American Journal of Preventive Medicine 10*(4), 217–222.

Drug and Alcohol Service Information System (DASIS) Report (2001). *Women in Substance Abuse Treatment*. DHHS: Washington, D.C.

Drug and Alcohol Service Information System (DASIS) Report (2002). *Black Admissions to Substance Abuse Treatment: 1999*. DHHS: Washington, D.C.

Friedman, S. R., Flom, P. L., Kottiri, B. J., Zenilman, J., Curtis, R., Neaigus, A., Sandoval, M., Quinn, T., & Des Jarlais, D. C. (2003). Drug use patterns and infection with sexually transmissible agents among young adults in a high-risk neighbourhood in New York City. *Addiction, 98*(2): 159–69.

Greenblatt, R. M., & Hessol, N. A. (2000). Epidemiology and natural history of HIV infection in women. In J. Anderson, (Ed.), A guide to the clinical care of women with HIV (pp. 1–33). Washington, DC: U.S. Dept. of Health and Human Services (HRSA): HIV/AIDS Division.

Hoffman, J. A., Klein, H., Clark, D. C., & Boyd, F. T. (1998). The effect of entering drug treatment on involvement in HIV-related risk behaviors. *American Journal of Drug and Alcohol Abuse, 24*, 259–284.

Holdaway, S. (1997) Some recent approaches to the study of race in criminological research. Race as social process. *The British Journal of Criminology, 37*, 383–400.

Institute of Medicine (2003). *Unequal Treatment: Confronting Racial & Ethnic Disparities in Health*. Portland, OR: National Academy Press.

Jansson, B. (1999). Becoming an effective policy advocate: From policy practice to social justice (3rd ed.). Pacific Grove: Brooks/Cole Publishing Company.

Joe, G. W., Simpson, D. D., & Broome, K. M. (1998). Effects of readiness for drug abuse treatment on client retention and assessment of process. *Addiction, 93*, 1177–1190.

Keigher, S., & Taylor-Brown, S. (2001). Women's health needs special treatment. *Health & Social Work, 26,* 67–71.

Land, H. (2000). AIDS and women of color. In V. J. Lynch. (Ed.), HIV/AIDS at year 2000: A sourcebook for social workers (pp. 79–96). Boston: Allyn and Bacon.

Longshore, D., Hsieh, S., & Anglin, M. D. (1993). Ethnic and gender differences in drug users' perceived need for treatment. *International Journal of the Addictions, 28(6),* 539–558.

MacMaster, S. A. (2005) Experiences and Perceptions of Barriers to Substance Abuse and HIV Service Access Among African American Women who use Crack Cocaine. *Journal of Ethnicity in Substance Abuse, 4,* (1), 53–75.

MacMaster, S. A., & Holleran, L. (2005). Incorporating 12-Step Group Attendance in Addictions Courses: An Experiential Cross-Cultural Experience. *Journal of Teaching in the Addictions, 4, (2).*

MacMaster, S. A., & Vail, K. V. (2002). Demystifying the Injection Drug User: Willingness to be involved in traditional drug treatment services among injection drug users involved in a needle exchange program. *Journal of Psychoactive Drugs, 34 (3),* 1–13.

Marx, R., Aral, S., Rolfs, R., Sterk, C., & Kahn, J. (1991). Crack, sex and STD. *Sexually Transmitted Diseases, 18,* 92–101.

Miller, W. R. & Rollnick, S. (1991). *Motivational Interviewing: Preparing People to Change Addictive Behavior.* New York: Guilford Press.

Morrow, K., & Allsworth, J. (2000). Sexual risk in lesbians and bisexual women. *Journal of Gay and Lesbian Medical Association, 4,* 159–165.

National Center for Health Statistics (NCHS). (2002). *Health, United States, 2002.* Hyattsville, Maryland: Public Health Service.

National Survey on Drug Use & Health (NSDUH). (2004). *2002: Latest National Survey on Drug Use & Health.* DHHS: Washington, D.C.

Needle, R. & Coyle, S. (1998). Community-based outreach risk-reduction strategy to prevent HIV risk behaviors in out-of-treatment injection drug users. In *NIH consensus development conference on interventions to prevent HIV risk behaviors. Program and abstracts* (pp. 81—87). Bethesda, MD: United States National Institutes of Health.

Parham, D., & Conviser, R. (2002). A brief history of the Ryan White CARE Act in the USA and its implications for other countries. *AIDS CARE, 14,* S3–S6.

Pequegnat, W., & Stover, E. (1999). Considering women's contextual and cultural issues in HIV/STD prevention research. *Cultural Diversity and Ethnic Minority Psychology, 5,* 287–291.

Prochaska, J. O., DiClemente, C. C., & Norcross, J. (1992). In search of how people change. *American Psychologist, 47,* 1102–1114.

Quinn, T. C. (1996). Global burden of the HIV pandemic. *Lancet, 348,* 99–106.

Ross, M., Ywang, L., Leonard, L., Teng, M., Duncan, L. (1999). Sexual behaviour, STDs, and drug use in a crack house population. *International Journal of STD and AIDS, 10,* 224–230.

Siplon, P. (2002). AIDS and the policy struggle in the United States. Washington, DC: Georgetown University Press.

Tennessee Department of Health (2002). *HIV/AIDS/STD Section Epidemiological Profile, 2001.* Nashville: Tennessee Department of Health

Treatment Data Episode Set (TEDS). (2004). Treatment Data Episode Set (TEDS) 1992–2001. DHHS: Washington, D.C.

U.S. Census Bureau. (2000, March). Poverty status of the population in 1999 by age, sex, and race and Hispanic origin. Washington, DC: Author.

Walton, E., Sandua-Beckler, P., & Mannes, M. (Eds.). (2001). Balancing family-centered services and child well-being: Exploring issues in policy, practice, theory and research. New York: Columbia University Press.

Wechsberg, W. M., Lam, W. K., Zule, W., Hall, G., Middlesteadt, R., & Edwards, J. (2003). Violence, homelessness, and HIV risk among crack-using African-American women. *Substance Use & Misuse, 38,* 671–701.

Wechsberg, W. M., Lam, W. K. K., Zule, W. A., & Bobashev, G. (2005). Efficacy of a woman-focused intervention to reduce HIV risk and increase self-sufficiency among African American crack abusers. *American Journal of Public Health, 94*(7): 1165–1173.

Wechsberg, W. M., W. Zule, R. Perritt, A. Roberts, R. Middlesteadt, and A. Burroughs (2001). "Women-Focused HIV Prevention for African-American Crack Users." In Harris, L.S. (Ed.), *Problems of Drug Dependence 2000: Proceedings of the 62nd Annual Scientific Meeting.* The College on Problems of Drug Dependence, Inc. NIDA Research Monograph 181, 2000. Bethesda, MD: US DHHS, pp. 33–34.

Wingood, G. M., & Di Clemente, R. J. (2000). The Willow program: Mobilizing social networks of women living with HIV to enhance coping and reduce sexual risk behaviors. In W. Pequegnat & J. Szapocznik (Eds.), Working with families in the era of HIV/AIDS (pp. 281–298). Thousand Oaks, CA: Sage Publications, Inc.

Wyatt, G. E., Moe, A., & Guthrie, D. (1999). The gynecological, reproductive, and sexual health of HIV-positive women. *Cultural Diversity and Ethnic Minority Psychology, 5,* 183–196.

Zule, W. A., Lam, W. K. K., & Wechsberg, W. M. (2003). "Treatment Readiness Among Out-of-Treatment African-American Crack Users." *Journal of Psychoactive Drugs, 35*(4).

HIV Prevention Programs in the Black Church: A Viable Health Promotion Resource for African American Women?

Schnavia Smith Hatcher
Jeronda T. Burley
Wilhelmena I. Lee-Ouga

The National Institute of Allergy and Infectious Diseases [NIAID], (2005) reported that, at the close of 2003, nearly 40 million people worldwide were living with the human immunodeficiency virus (HIV), which is the virus that causes acquired immunodeficiency syndrome (AIDS). The organization also reported that since identification in 1981, AIDS has claimed the lives of more than 20 million people (NI-

AID). Men and women of all races have been affected by HIV/AIDS since the first cases were reported. However, women and people of color have experienced the greatest rates of infection. Women account for more than 50% of the existing 40 million HIV/AIDS cases to date (Centers for Disease Control and Prevention [CDCP], 2004). Moreover, according to the CDCP (2004), African-American women are infected with HIV/AIDS 25 times more often than white women and four times more often than Hispanic women, making HIV/AIDS the leading cause of death for Black women ages 25–34.

Currently, there is no cure for HIV/AIDS, and the only certain way to prevent the spread of HIV/AIDS is abstinence, which means to abstain from sexual intercourse. Besides abstinence, the use of condoms is an effective means of prohibiting the transmission of the virus (CDCP, 2004). When used correctly and consistently, latex or polyurethane condoms offer the greatest barrier to HIV. However, the sole recommendation of condom use is inadequate, as evidenced by the rates of HIV infection among African-American women. The findings point to the importance of rethinking current approaches to promoting condom use in prevention programs that target this population.

Schiele (1996) noted that persons within the African Diaspora have experienced decades of destruction and oppression, which continue to impact the lives of people of color. More recently, the devastation of HIV disease has served to further decimate a nation of people both nationally and internationally (Butler, 1997; Moore, Madison-Colmore, & Moore, 2003; Schiele, 1996; Schiele, 2000). Paradigms such as Afrocentricity, black psychology, and black pastoral psychology provide a needed cultural response to the copious struggles that particularly plague these communities of color.

Given the increasing rate of transmission with this population, the purpose of this article is to review the existing literature to investigate the risk factors associated with African-American women with HIV/AIDS and identify an effective method of HIV prevention for them. The literature review will include an investigation of factors such as gender-related prevention concerns and cultural relevant prevention issues. A discussion of religion and African-Americans in terms of the Black church and its health promotion efforts will also be included. The article concludes with a discussion of program elements of HIV prevention programs in the Black church and possible challenges faced for the programs. Recommendations for future research to improve service provisions for the population will also be provided.

THE INFLUENCE OF GENDER AND
CULTURAL-SPECIFIC RISK FACTORS

The impact of HIV risk factors can vary among men and women. Likewise, aspects related to culture are also distinct. For this reason, research suggests that HIV prevention efforts be gender-specific and cultural-related in order to address gender role perceptions that have helped to promote the spread of the virus (Gasch, Poulson, Fullilove, & Fullilove, 1991; Kelly, 1995).

For women, the primary mode of HIV transmission is through heterosexual contact with an HIV-infected partner (NIAID, 2005). NIAID (2005) reported that women in the United States have a greater chance than men of contracting HIV from an infected partner through heterosexual intercourse. Markedly, exposure to substantial amounts of seminal fluids and ulcerations in the vagina caused by sexually transmitted infections (STIs) contribute to women's increased risk of HIV disease.

In addition to sexual activity, studies show that a high prevalence of substance abuse exists among women with HIV (Brems, Fisher, & Queen, 1998; El-Bassel, Witte, Wada, Gilbert, & Wallace, 2001). Research suggests that occupational factors lead some women (i.e., commercial sex workers) to use drugs and alcohol as a coping mechanism to deal with the daily stressors of their work environment (El-

Bassel et al., 2001). Using HIV-contaminated needles or syringes also contributes to high rates of HIV infection among women (El-Bassel, et al., 2001). Though the relationship between HIV and substance abuse is well known, many health care providers fail to provide drug-using women HIV information during office visits (Brems et al.). These findings are important and dictate that prevention efforts for women must continue to address the intersection of these public health concerns.

Another important factor for clinicians to consider regarding substance-abusing women and correlates to HIV is the likelihood of experienced partner violence. According to El-Bassel et al. (2001), the stigma associated with being a female drug addict often leads to partner violence and possible conflicts over condom use. Women who have been a victim of violence will probably present with anal, genital, and nongenital trauma, which subsequently increases the risk of HIV transmission. Also, abused women are more likely to have an STI, which provides an additional opportunity for the spread of HIV (Brems, Fisher, & Queen, 1998; El-Bassel et al., 1998). Because this population does not have regular access to health care, many of these HIV risk factors may go unnoticed by health care providers.

Psychiatric comorbidities, such as depression, anxiety and posttraumatic stress disorder, have also been found to be associated with HIV-risk sexual behaviors and injecting drug use among women (CDCP, 2004). Traditional outreach programs providing substance abuse and HIV-related services for this population frequently are challenged in their attempts to meet the comprehensive client care needs associated with HIV infection, high-risk behaviors, and psychiatric comorbidities. This research, again, substantiates the need for health care providers to become more involved in HIV prevention, especially where it concerns women.

Other studies that examined HIV risk factors commonly found among African-American women discovered that denial of HIV risk was extremely prevalent (Crosby, Yarber, DiClemente, Wingood, & Meyerson, 2002; Sobo, 1993; Timmons & Sowell, 1999). Women who felt safe in their relationships reported inconsistent condom use or no condom use at all because for some black women, condoms reportedly represent a lack of love, trust, and commitment (Crosby et al., 2002). The CDC (2004) also reported that some women experience fear of abuse or abandonment in relationships, which inhibits them from requiring their male partner to use condoms. Condoms use is effective in preventing the spread of HIV infection and should be encouraged, but in conjunction with a more complete HIV prevention message that also includes condom negotiation techniques and sexual assertiveness (CDC, 2004).

Many studies stress the importance of developing culturally appropriate HIV prevention programs in order to reduce the HIV/AIDS rates among African-Americans (DeMarco & Norris, 2004; Gasch et al., 1991; Moore et al., 2003; Schiele, 1996; Vinh-Thomas, Bunch, & Card, 2003; Wilson & Miller, 2003). These studies have highlighted Afrocentric approaches, such as Afrocentricity, black psychology, black pastoral psychology, as viable alternatives to traditional Eurocentric approaches used to explain African-American behavior and thereby direct the development of HIV prevention programs (Butler, 1997; Moore et al., 2003; Schiele, 1996). The paradigms guide approaches that place special emphasis on culture and history in order to give credence to the experiences of people of African descent (Moore et al., 2003; Schiele, 1996). Specifically, Afrocentric approaches acknowledge the impact of experiences among black people through its incorporation into prevention strategies. For example, Gasch et al. (1991) suggest a three-pronged approach to HIV prevention for the African-American community. First, addressing and positively reframing the widely held genocidal conspiracy held by many African-Americans is imperative. Second, the influence of gender roles on the spread of HIV must be acknowledged. Finally, HIV prevention programs should address the impact of ecological decline on communities of color. By incorporating an Afrocentric perspective, HIV strategies are likely to be more inclusive and relevant to the issues faced by African-American people (Butler, 1997; Moore et al., 2003; Schiele, 1996).

HIV PREVENTION IN THE BLACK CHURCH: A PRACTICAL PREVENTION STRATEGY

Studies consistently report a decrease in high-risk sexual behavior for African-American women participating in comprehensive HIV prevention programs that include multiple sessions focusing on behavioral skills and reduction of risk behavior (Eldridge et al., 1997; Robinson et al., 2002). Additional research confirms that programs with individual and community-level interventions focusing on the social context of African-American women are most likely to reduce high risk behavior than programs that only provide HIV information (Dancy, Marcantonio, & Norr, 2000; Kelly, 1995; Lauby, Smith, Stark, Person, & Adams, 2000; Luckey, 1995; Marlow, West, Corrigan, Pena,

& Cunningham, 1994; Sikkema, Kelly, Winett, Solomon, Cargill, & Roffman, 2000). Therefore, a comprehensive program addressing both cultural knowledge and behavior—in particular, a faith-based organization in the community—seems to be a viable option for HIV prevention programs targeting African-American women.

Religiosity

Researchers commonly define religiosity in terms of public behavior that consists of the frequency of church attendance and private behavior, a person's devotional or prayer time (Davidson, Darling, & Norton, 1995; Davidson, Moore, & Ullstrup, 2004; Fehring, Cheever, German, & Philpot, 1998; Morse, Morse, Klebra, Stock, Forehand, & Panayotova, 2000). Religion remains an integral part of African-American culture and tends to permeate every aspect of black life (Schiele, 2000). Furthermore, women are more likely than men to deem religion as important and to demonstrate their commitment by attending religious services on a weekly basis (Pew Research Center for the People & the Press, 2001). On the basis of data from the General Survey from 1992 to 2002, Wilcox (2005) indicated that weekly religious attendance rates for black women are higher than for white and Latina women and higher than men, regardless of race. Wolk (2006) noted that the relationship between black women and religion is one that has changed over time and from one organization to another; though still considered low in number and support, nationwide, black females now account for approximately 3% of clergy.

As indicated, religion is an essential part of African-American culture. The Black church is one of the most stable institutions in the African-American community (Billingsley & Caldwell, 1991; Douglas and Hopson, 2001; Lincoln & Mamiya, 1990; Schiele, 2000). Douglas and Hopson defined the Black church as "a multitudinous community of churches, which are diversified by origin, denomination, doctrine, worshipping culture, spiritual expression, class, size, and other less obvious factors ... they share a special history, culture, and role in Black life, all of which attest to their collective identity as the Black church" (p. 96). It is the place where most black persons celebrate their faith and seek direction.

In that vein, studies have indicated that religiosity has been consistently found to be a predictor of sexual behavior among adolescents, college students, and adult women (Davidson, Darling, & Norton,

1995; Elifson, Klein, & Sterk, 2003; Fehring et al., 1998; Morse et al., 2000). Specifically, persons who frequently attend religious services or report consistent devotional time have fewer high-risk sexual behaviors and delays in first sexual intercourse experience. Historically, the Black church has represented an instrument of social justice and a place of political mobilization and community awareness (Billingsley & Caldwell, 1991; Newlin, Knafl, & Melkus, 2002; Pattillo-McCoy, 1998). Therefore, it is implicit that HIV prevention conducted within a religious setting, such as the Black church, would be effective in reducing HIV among communities of color.

The Black Church and Health Promotion

The role of the Black church in health promotion and HIV prevention is not a recent effort. However, it is a role that is still being defined and enhanced. Several studies note that African-Americans have historically utilized their church or minister as a resource on a variety of health-related topics, such as hypertension, stroke, and diabetes (Aaron, Levine, & Burstin, 2003; Elifson et al., 2003; Taylor, Ellison, Chatters, Levin, & Lincoln, 2000; Williams, Griffith, Young, Collins, & Dodson, 1999). Scholars have also found that church outreach programs have substantial participation by its membership and the community, perhaps owing to the fact that most of these programs are offered free of charge and are conducted by trusted and well-respected individuals of faith (Taylor et al., 2000; Thomas et al., 1991; Williams et al., 1999).

Predictors for Health Promotion Programs. Several researchers agree that congregation size is a key predictor for Black churches with health promotion programs (Taylor et al., 2000; Thomas et al., 1994). Studies suggest that larger congregations tend to have greater resources than congregations with fewer members; numerous volunteers and paid staff are typically available to large congregations (Taylor et al., 2000; Williams et al., 1999). The second greatest predictor of the church's involvement in health promotion is the minister. Research indicates that the minister's support, educational level, and level of service delivery collectively predict the development and tenure of faith-based programs (Ammerman et al., 2003; Ellison, Chatters, Levin, & Lincoln, 2000; Griffith, Young, Collins, & Dodson, 1999).

Types of Health Promotion. As mentioned previously, black churches have successfully implemented various types of health promotion programs, such as hypertension, mental health, drug prevention, and social support (Krause, Ellison, Shaw, Marcum, & Boardman, 2001; Smith & Merritt, 1997; Taylor et al., 2000). In fact, Lincoln & Mamiya (1990) found that Black churches operate community-based programs more often than do white churches. Therefore, the Black church's efforts to develop HIV prevention programs targeting the African-American community are not surprising or unforeseen.

HIV Health Promotion. Faith-based HIV prevention programs are emerging steadily, especially as eligible government funding becomes available. However, evaluation outcomes remain limited, causing some to withhold confidence in HIV prevention programs conducted by faith-based organizations (i.e. churches, temples, and synagogues). Some feel that religious doctrine might hinder faith-based organizations from providing effective HIV/AIDS prevention services (Coleman, 2004; Fullilove & Fullilove, 1999; Lemell, 2004). Consequently, the HIV/AIDS epidemic in the African-American community has forced faith-based organizations, the Black church specifically, to reexamine its doctrinal beliefs in order to determine how best to respond to this health crisis. The result of this religious critique has been the development of HIV prevention programs by Black churches, substantial research examining the Black church and its prevention efforts, and federal funding for which faith-organizations are eligible.

Program Elements of HIV Prevention in the Black Church

Balm in Gilead, Inc. is a leader in the education and engagement of African-American clergy across the nation in an effort to increase their involvement in HIV prevention and treatment for members of their churches and communities (Balm in Gilead, 2006). Specifically, Balm in Gilead promotes, organizes and integrates HIV/AIDS awareness and outreach activities into the ministries of Black churches. For example, its Black Church HIV/AIDS Training Institute convenes African-American HIV/AIDS experts to train black pastors and church members on the biological, psychosocial, and economic factors associated with AIDS in the black community. The Institute's curriculum is designed to promote an understanding of Biblical scripture to support church involvement in social activism and personal ministries to individuals infected and affected by HIV/AIDS. The curriculum includes skill-building courses to integrate AIDS knowledge into counseling, outreach, and numerous other aspects of church life. Other Balm in Gilead activities include The Black Church Week of Prayer for the

Healing of AIDS, which encourages black congregations to address the HIV/AIDS epidemic from the pulpit (it suggests prayers and projects to focus members' thoughts and activities around the AIDS crisis in the black community); The Church Lights the Way: HIV Testing Campaign; and a Faith-Based HIV/AIDS Technical Assistance Center (Balm in Gilead).

In a similar effort to convene black faith leaders around a common concern about AIDS in the black community, the California Statewide HIV/AIDS Church Outreach Advisory Board and the California Department of Health Services, Office of AIDS collaborated to increase awareness and educate congregations on ways to participate in the prevention of HIV transmission (Black News, 2006). Promotion of National HIV Testing Days, HIV-related topical discussion groups, and sermons to stir compassion for individuals impacted by the AIDS epidemic are among their activities. In addition, the Board designed and subsequently distributed thousands of copies of a resource for pastors titled "Healing Begins Here: A Pastor's Guidebook to HIV/AIDS Ministry through the Church" (Black News, 2006).

While these programs exemplify targeted efforts to address the HIV/AIDS epidemic directly, other Black church activities have addressed determinants of HIV by turning their focus to the topic of sexuality in the church. Most notably, the Religious Coalition for Reproductive Choice (2006) spawned the National Black Church Initiative in 1996. The Initiative sponsors an annual National Black Religious Summit on Sexuality that promotes dialogue between clergy and laity on issues such as teen pregnancy, sexuality and religion, domestic violence, reproductive health, and HIV/AIDS. In addition, "Keeping It Real," "Hear Me Now," and "Breaking the Silence" are discussion tools/curricula it promotes that address sexuality education for teens and families (Religious Coalition for Reproductive Choice, 2006). While some proponents of HIV/AIDS education in the church have voiced concern that these curricula solely promote an abstinence-only prevention model, this formalization of sexuality education in the Black church represents an increased awareness that remaining silent about the risk factors of HIV/AIDS is no longer acceptable (Religious Coalition for Reproductive Choice, 2006; Veazey, 2005).

These programs, though impressive in their proactive design to move the Black church into greater acknowledgement, understanding and involvement regarding HIV/AIDS prevention activities, lack systematic evidence of impact or outcome effectiveness at this time. To gain a better understanding of the effect that church-based HIV prevention programs have on desired changes in the perceptions, attitudes, and behaviors believed pertinent to reducing HIV risks among black women, systematic, wide-spread diffusion of innovative programs must occur (Rogers, 1995). Yet, it is noteworthy to mention that employing the diffusion of innovations theory would support the observed reality that new ideas and innovative approaches such as Black church-sponsored HIV health promotion move slowly throughout the society.

Challenges with HIV Prevention in the Black Church

While the movement grows to involve Black church leaders and their members in the fight against HIV/AIDS, engagement of local congregations across the nation is not yet the norm. Though some research implies that the future may hold greater openness to HIV health promotion, a number of factors inherent in Black church culture and associated religious doctrine challenge the acceptance of many tenets of HIV health promotion commonly utilized in secular settings.

Early in the second decade of the epidemic, a survey of black clergy revealed that more than three-fourths of sermons preached on sexuality were against premarital sex (79%) and/or included unwavering opposition to homosexuality (Anderson, 2000). Anderson also reported that in another survey of ministers attending the 1992 Hampton University Ministers Conference, more than one-third (35%) of respondents believed HIV/AIDS is a curse from God. In contrast, nearly a decade later, a similar survey of ministers revealed that a majority of respondents believed that HIV/AIDS was among the top issues in which the Black church should be involved (Harris, 2000). This change in beliefs has been slow to translate into behavior change that embraces a religious agenda inclusive of HIV health outreach ministry. Thus, conservative beliefs and attitudes about HIV risk factors continue to permeate Black church culture leading individual church members who may desire to engage in HIV health promotion activities to instead experience conflict between their conviction to help and their concern regarding potential stigmatization.

Conversely, Mackie Norris, an expert on the relationship between religion and health and a noted leader in the United Methodist Church, similarizes the presentation of HIV disease to a threat to civil rights. Norris asserted that this analogy necessitates a familiar response of the Black church to act as a liberating institution consistent not only with its civil rights movement history but with New Testament examples of response to suffering. According to Norris, the New Testament confronts suffering at both the systems level and the personal level. In the AIDS epidemic, the systems level calls federal, state, and local governments and related systems to provide resources, attitudes and an environment in which the HIV/AIDS epidemic can be addressed (Norris, 1995). The personal level relieves the physical, mental and emotional suffering of those afflicted with the disease (Norris, 1995). In that manner, the national presidents of the Women's Missionary Society of the African Methodist Episcopal Church, the African Methodist Episcopal Zion Church, and Christian Methodist Episcopal Church have partnered with the Balm In Gilead, Inc. to build the capacity of these denominations to address HIV/AIDS and other health disparities among black people (Balm in Gilead, 2006). This partnership is also designed to build a sustainable health education and service delivery system within African-American faith communities.

Notwithstanding the increased number of voices acknowledging the legitimacy and need for Black church leadership and involvement in HIV programs, it is acknowledged that proven measures of outcome effectiveness are often lacking in such endeavors to date. Some exception may exist among faith-based HIV organizations that receive federal funding through the Substance Abuse and Mental Health Services Administration (SAMHSA), for example. These faith-based HIV programs are required to track and report on specific National Outcome Measures (NOMS). Similarly, programs funded through the CDC report on outcomes that are summarized in the annual HIV/AIDS Surveillance Report. However, such data submitted for national compilation typically are not utilized to determine the effectiveness of local programs or programmatic components. That is, a clear linkage between client- or organizational-level outcomes observed and program/service delivery components implemented is most often not established.

While federally-funded programs may offer a base from which to expand evaluation practices of faith-based organizations, an additional concern presents in that many faith-based programs do not receive federal funding due to a number of perceived barriers that deter many religious organizations from seeking federal support. Though the promise of change exists in the current political climate, federal funding historically has been accompanied by restrictions on religious activities, such as denial of faith-based organizations' choice to consider religion in hiring decisions, complicated application processes, cumbersome grant agreements, and slow funding reimbursements, for examples (Independent Sector, 2004). Thus, a need exists for increased availability of training opportunities in program evaluation, user-friendly evaluation tools, and ongoing program evaluation coaching for clergy and laity that seek to provide HIV prevention programs in the Black Church. Also needed is an increase of funding mechanisms with grant application requirements and conditions of award that are not prohibitive to small and/or medium-sized church/faith-based organizations which are likely to have access to populations in need of HIV prevention services.

CONCLUSION

African-American women experience a disproportionate burden of the HIV/AIDS epidemic, in terms of experienced risk factors for HIV and the resulting incidence and prevalence of HIV/AIDS cases. In tandem, Black church membership in the United States is predominantly female. Thus, the rationale for greater involvement in HIV outreach, prevention, and related public health activities among Black churches and the beneficial impact on their involvement on women is discernible.

Currently, though Black church–based HIV prevention program models exist, a more rapid increase in the numbers of similar programs is hindered by perceived conflicts between doctrinal beliefs and a need to embrace individuals whose lifestyle behaviors may contradict religious standards and Black church culture. Continued education, dialogue, and persistent effort to promote a scriptural rationale for attending to the needs of all who are sick and afflicted in the black community is likely to result in increased willingness of the Black church to provide outreach to those who suffer directly and indirectly from HIV and AIDS.

In spite of the wealth of information on African-American women and HIV prevention, the existing body of research is lacking information on model HIV prevention programs conducted in religious settings. It is recommended that existing religiously affiliated HIV prevention programs begin to conduct program evaluations in order to populate the research base of faith-based interventions. It is also tendered that replicable models of faith-based HIV prevention programs be developed. Furthermore, HIV prevention research on African-American women needs to be expanded in order to include other socioeconomic groups. Much of recent data maintains drug-using, low-income women or college students as the primary target populations of most HIV prevention studies. There is limited HIV prevention research available on middle-class African-American, non-substance-abusing women at risk for HIV/AIDS.

The debate regarding the promotion of HIV prevention programs for African-American women in the Black church will persist. However, AIDS is now the number one cause of death for Black adults aged 25–44, before heart disease, cancer and homicide (CDCP, 2004). As social work professionals working in the community, we must continue with our roles as broker, liaison, and case manager of services for our clients and facilitate health promotion that will decrease the rapidly increasing percentage of HIV/AIDS cases for this population. As noted, a relatively few innovators have initiated church-based HIV health promotion activities that are likely to influence additional churches to adopt similar practices over time. Strategic information sharing will help promote understanding of the benefits and manage uncertainty to effect social change around the critical need for new venues, such as the Black church, to reach black women and their families impacted by the multiple facets of the HIV/AIDS epidemic.

REFERENCES

Aaron, K., Levine, D., & Burstin, H. (2003). African American church participation and health care practice. *Journal of General Internal Medicine, 18*, 908–913.

Ammerman, A., Corbie-Smith, G., St. George, D. M., Washington, C., Weathers, B., & Jackson-Christian, B. (2003). Research expectations among African American church leaders in the PRAISE project: A randomized trial guided by community-based participatory research. *American Journal of Public Health, 19*(10), 1720–1727.

Anderson, V. (2000). The black church and sexual ethics. Retrieved March 5, 2006, from http://www.clgs.org/5/black_church_sexual_ethics.html

Balm in Gilead. (2006). Programs of the balm. Retrieved March 1, 2006, from http://www.balmingilead.org/programs

Billingsley, A., & Caldwell, C. (1991). The church, the family, and the school in the African American community. *Journal of Negro Education, 60*(3), 427–440.

Black News. (2006). Black Church Leaders Gather to Develop A Faith-Based Strategy to Prevent HIV and AIDS. Retrieved April 16, 2006 from http://www.blacknews.com/pr/blackchurchleaders101.html.

Brems, C., Fisher, D., & Queen, P. (1998). Physicians' assessment of drug use and other HIV risk behavior: Reports by female drug users. *Drugs and Society, 13*(1–2), 145–159.

Bulter, L. (1997). African American pastoral psychology in the twenty-first century will be more than sensual healing. *Journal of Religious Thought, 53/54*(2-1), 113–121.

Centers for Disease Control and Prevention. (2004). *Fact sheet: HIV/AIDS among women.* Atlanta, GA: Author.

Coleman, C. (2004). The contribution of religious and existential well-being to depression among African American depression among African American heterosexuals with HIV infection. *Issues in Mental Health Nursing, 25,* 103–110.

Crosby, R., Yarber, W., DiClemente, R., Wingood, G., & Meyerson, B. (2002). HIV-associated histories, perceptions, and practices among low-income African American women: Does rural residence matter? *American Journal of Public Health, 92*(4), 655–659.

Dancy, B., Marcantonio, R., & Norr, K. (2000). The long-term effectiveness of an HIV prevention intervention for low-income African American women. *AIDS Education and Prevention, 12*(2), 113–125.

Davidson, C., Darling, C., & Norton, L. (1995). Religiosity and the sexuality of women: Sexual behavior and sexual satisfaction revisited. *Journal of Sex Research, 32*(3), 235–244.

Davidson, J., Moore, N., & Ullstrup, K. (2004). Religiosity and sexual responsibility: Relationships of choice. *American Journal of Health Behavior, 28*(4), 335–346.

DeMarco, R., & Norris, A. (2004). Culturally relevant HIV interventions: Transcending ethnicity. *Journal of Cultural Diversity, 11*(2), 65–68.

Douglas, K., & Hopson, R. (2001). Understanding the Black church: Dynamics of change. *Journal of Religious Thought, 56/57*(2-1), 95–113.

El-Bassel, N., Gilbert, L., Krishnan, S., Schilling, R., Gaeta, T., & Purpura, S. (1998). Partner violence and sexual HIV-risk behaviors among women in an inner-city emergency department. *Violence and Victims, 13*(4), 377–393.

El-Bassel, N., Witte, S., Wada, T., Gilbert, L., & Wallace, J. (2001). Correlates of partner violence among female street-based sex workers: Substance abuse, history, of childhood abuse, and HIV risks. *AIDS Patient Care and STDs, 15,* 41–51.

Eldridge, G., St. Lawrence, J., Little, C., Shelby, M., Brasfield, T., & Service, J. (1997). Evaluation of an HIV risk reduction intervention for women entering inpatient substance abuse treatment. *AIDS Education and Prevention, 9*(1), 62–76.

Elifson, K., Klein, H., & Sterk, C. (2003). Religiosity and HIV risk behavior involvement among "at risk" women. *Journal of Religion and Health, 42*(1), 47–66.

Fehring, R., Cheever, K., German, K., & Philpot, C. (1998). Religiosity and sexual activity among older adolescents. *Journal of Religion and Health, 37*(3), 229–247.

Fullilove, M., & Fullilove, R. (1999). Stigma as an obstacle to AIDS action. *The American Behavioral Scientist, 42*(7), 1117–1129.

Gasch, H., Poulson, M., Fullilove, R., & Fullilove, M. (1991). Shaping AIDS education and prevention programs for African Americans amidst community decline. *The Journal of Negro Education, 60*(1), 85–96.

Harris, H. (2000, July 22). Sins, sermons and sexuality: New attitude of openness found in poll of pastors. *The Washington Post,* p. B9.

Independent Sector. (2004). Unlevel Playing Field: Barriers to Participation by Faith-Based and Community Organizations in Federal Social Service Programs. Retrieved on July 24, 2006, from http://www.independentsector.org.

Kelly, J. (1995). Advances in HIV/AIDS education and prevention. *Family Relations,* *44*(4), 345–352.

Krause, N., Ellison, C., Shaw, B., Marcum, J., & Boardman, J. (2001). Church-based social support and religious coping. *Journal for the Scientific Study of Religion,* *40*(4), 637–656.

Lauby, J., Smith, P., Stark, M., Person, B., & Adams, J. (2000). A community-level HIV prevention intervention for inner-city women: Results of the women and infants demonstration projects. *American Journal of Public Health, 90*(2), 216–222.

Lemell, A. (2004). African American attitudes toward gay males: Faith-based initiatives and implications for HIV/AIDS services. *Journal of African American Studies, 7*(4), 59–74.

Lincoln, C., & Mamiya, L. (1990). *The Black church in the African American experience.* Durham, NC: Duke University Press.

Luckey, I. (1995). HIV/AIDS prevention in the African American community: An integrated community-based practice approach. *Journal of Community Practice,* *2*(4), 71–90.

Marlow, R. M., West, J. A., Corrigan, S. A., Pena, J. M., & Cunningham, S. (1994). Outcome of psychoeducation for HIV risk reduction. *AIDS Education and Prevention, 6*(2), 113–125.

Moore, S., Madison-Colmore, O., & Moore, J. (2003). An Afrocentric approach to substance abuse treatment with adolescent African American males: Two case examples. *The Western Journal of Black Studies, 27*(4), 219–230.

Morse, E., Morse, P., Klebra, K., Stock, M., Forehand, R., & Panayotova, E. (2000). The use of religion among HIV-infected African American women. *Journal of Religion and Health, 39*(3), 261–276.

National Institute of Allergy and Infectious Diseases (NIAID). (2005). HIV infection in women. Retrieved April 21, 2005, from http://www.niaid.nih.gov/factsheets/womenhiv.htm

Newlin, K., Knafl, K., & Melkus, G. (2002). African American spirituality: A concept analysis. *Advances in Nursing Science, 25*(2), 57–70.

Norris, M. (1995). *The Black Church and the AIDS Crisis, Focus paper #29.* New York: Health and Welfare Ministries, General Board of Global Ministries, United Methodist Church.

Pattillo-McCoy, M. (1998). Church culture as a strategy of action in the Black community. *American Sociological Review, 63*(12), 767–784.

Pew Research Center for the People & the Press. (2001). Survey Reports: Religion in American Life. Retrieved on April 12, 2006, from http://people-press.org/reports.

Religious Coalition for Reproductive Choice (2006). Black Church Initiative. Retrieved April 20, 2006 from http://www.rcrc.org/programs/blackchurch.cfm.

Robinson, B., Uhl, G., Miner, M., Bockting, W., Scheltema, K., Rosser, B. R., et al. (2002). Evaluation of a sexual health approach to prevent HIV among low income, urban, primarily African American women: Results of a randomized controlled trial. *AIDS Education and Prevention, 14*(Suppl A), 81–96.

Rogers, E. (1995). *Diffusion of innovations,* 4th ed. New York: The Free Press.

Schiele, J. (1996). Afrocentricity: An emerging paradigm in social work practice. *Social Work, 41*(3), 284–295.

Schiele, J. (2000). *Human services and the Afrocentric paradigm.* New York: The Haworth Press.

Sikkema, K., Kelly, J., Winett, R., Solomon, L., Cargill, V., & Roffman, R. (2001). Outcomes of a randomized community-level HIV prevention intervention for women living in 18 low-income housing developments. *American Journal of Public Health, 90*(1), 57–63.

Smith, E., & Merritt, S. (1997). Church-based education: An outreach program for African Americans with hypertension. *Ethnicity and Health, 2*(3), 24–38.

Sobo, E. (1993). Inner-city women and AIDS: The psycho-social benefits of unsafe sex. *Culture, Medicine, and Psychiatry, 17*, 455–485.

Taylor, R., Ellison, C., Chatters, L., Levin, J., & Lincoln, K. (2000). Mental health services in faith communities: The role of clergy in Black churches. *Social Work, 45*(1), 73–87.

Thomas, S., Quinn, S., Billingsley, A., & Caldwell C. (1994). The characteristics of northern Black churches with community health outreach programs. *American Journal of Public Health, 84*(4), 575–579.

Timmons, S., & Sowell, R. (1999). Perceived HIV-related sexual risks and prevention practices of African American women in the southeastern United States. *Health Care for Women International, 20*, 579–591.

Veazey, C. (2005). *Faith-based sexuality education breaks the silence in black churches.* Norwalk, CT: Religious Institute on Sexual Morality, Justice, and Healing.

Vinh-Thomas, P., Bunch, M., & Card, J. (2003). A research-based tool for identifying and strengthening culturally competent and evaluation-ready HIV/AIDS prevention programs. *AIDS Education and Prevention, 15*(6), 481–498.

Williams, D., Griffith, E., Young, J., Collins, C., & Dodson, J. (1999). Structure and provision of services in Black churches in New Haven, CT. *Cultural Diversity and Ethnic Minority Psychology, 5*(2), 118–133.

Wilcox, W. (2005). Analysis: Religion, family, and the general social survey. Retrieved February 1, 2005, from http://www.pbs.org/wnet/religionandethics/week908/analysis1.

Wilson, B., & Miller, R. (2003). Examining strategies for culturally grounded HIV prevention: A review. *AIDS Education and Prevention, 15*(2), 184–202.

Wolk, B. (2006) Women and the church-North America: American Baptist women ministries. Retrieved March 1, 2006, from http://dickinsg.intrasun.tcnj.edu/diaspora/women.html

Women, Economic Development, and HIV/AIDS: Transforming Systems of Care for Sustainable Change

Lisa M. Webb-Robins
Na'ama Ben David

It is estimated that 28% of people (more than 5.3 million) in South Africa have been affected by HIV/AIDS, and more than 13% of all the people in the world living with HIV can be found in that country (UNAIDS, 2004). These statistics, along with a multitude of others, give evidence to suggest that not only is HIV/AIDS an epidemic that has reached crisis proportions but that it particularly invades economically depressed and poverty-stricken areas across the world. HIV/AIDS is considered to be one of six diseases of poverty by the World Health Organization, along with tuberculosis, malaria, measles, pneumonia, and diarrheal disease (WHO, 2005). These specific diseases are so named owing to the fact that they primarily affect the poor, they worsen poverty's toll, and they can generally be treated for a small amount of money. The overall economic losses suffered by victims and their families lead to a substantial economic strain on already depleted community and national resources.

The impact of HIV/AIDS on women is particularly profound. A recent report produced by the UN Population Fund (2005) indicates that nearly 60% of present HIV/AIDS infections are in women, with young women aged between 15 and 24 being at least three times more likely to be HIV-positive than men of the same age range. UNAIDS reports that "among women surveyed in Harare (Zimbabwe), Durban and Soweto (South Africa), 66 percent reported having one lifetime partner, 79 percent had abstained from sex at least until the age of 17 ... yet 40 percent of the young women were HIV-positive" (UNAIDS, 2005). Of further concern, women who are financially dependent on their male partner find it difficult to negotiate the use of condoms or to refuse unprotected sex even if they suspect their partner is infected or sick. The victimization of these women does not end with the deprioritization of their own physical health and well-being. Most often, when the husband and primary breadwinner becomes sick, most of the responsibility of caring for him, as well as other infected family members, falls on the women.

Throughout the world, there are a variety of approaches utilized for both the prevention and treatment of HIV/AIDS. In South Africa, however, the most emphasis is put on the use of antiretroviral (ARV) and combination pharmaceutical therapies as the treatment course in the wake of failed prevention approaches (De Cock, 2002). Most South African HIV/AIDS clinics prioritize the biological aspects of the virus (Singh, Berman, Swindells, et al., 1999) with psychosocial consequences of the AIDS epidemic in Africa having been less documented (Evans et al., 1997; Greenfield et al., 1997; Uys, 2002). There is scarce documentation surrounding the psychosocial aspects of the illness, suicide, and resultant loss of hope (Baingana, Thomas,

& Comblain, 2005). The connection between body and mind in both prevention and management is largely ignored.

Generally, in industrialized nations, the link between psychological and physiological health is well documented. In extreme stress situations, psychological and physiological systems deteriorate, resulting in compromised immunity and increased susceptibility to illness. Persons living with HIV/AIDS (PLWHA) face a number of significant psychological stressors such as extreme poverty, malnutrition, and stigma (Wessels, van Kredenburg, Aronson, Wilson, & Stein, 1998) that can lead to decreased physiological resiliency, thus hindering the goals of primary care and antiretroviral therapies. The WHO asserts that the mental health consequences of AIDS are "substantial" (WHO, 2004) with general emotional responses of "anger, guilt, fear, denial, and despair" being ever present (Gallego, Gordillo, & Catalan, 2000). Despite an exhaustive search, the authors were unable to find any program in existence that holistically addresses issues present in PLWHA. Therefore, the need for a holistic system that addresses multiple layers of care of the person is evident. The traditional "one size fits all" approach surrounding ARV treatment is simply not meeting the socioeconomic needs of economically depressed corners of the world.

It has been proposed (World Health Organization, 2001) that "treatment is not just a moral necessity, but a necessary component of economic stabilization and an ultimate return to economic development in high prevalence parts of the world." Two treatment approaches that have received only a modicum of attention to date but are emerging as significant considerations involve the aspects of employment and sociological health in HIV-positive individuals and their resultant impacts upon the workplace and economic development in developing countries. However, acknowledgment of the need for these kinds of interdependent approaches becomes apparent in social subtext. Recently, the World Bank (2005) issued a statement regarding HIV/AIDS care planning:

> HIV/AIDS *planning tends to be poor*: too little planning (in the rush to apply for funding and then spend it), too many plans (to please a variety of donors) with very little coordination, and an inability to plan effectively (especially at the national level). . . . This results in misallocated funds and little chance of impact; in one country only 1 percent of program resources target the particular risk groups that cause 75 percent of new infections." (World Bank)

The proposal of a larger systems approach to treatment of HIV/ AIDS would be a strategy that encompasses multiple layers of care. These layers would take a strategic approach that evaluates the economic factors present in a country with considerable HIV infection rates as well as the biological treatment issues to look at the long range sustainability of interventions. It would be similar to an approach that takes kindling and puts it on a fire (focused initiative with long-term potential) as opposed to pouring gasoline (many donor funds that are quickly exhausted) that will satisfy a few but dwindle to only ashes with no source for renewal. With this as a primary consideration, the authors raise the factor of "work" for those who have HIV, the related psychological change that is associated with employment and the concept of employment as a part of a comprehensive overall treatment approach for HIV-positive individuals.

In this concept article, the authors utilize Maslow's Hierarchy to define a proposed conceptual treatment framework that includes economic development efforts and discuss examples of successes that have been demonstrated in the literature. The authors posit that HIV/ AIDS treatment practitioners should not overlook the interconnectedness and interdependency of economic equilibrium and public health and suggest that the creation of treatment plans based on multidimensional interdisciplinary approaches are necessary to achieve maximum benefit for care and resource dollars.

HEALTH NEEDS AND MASLOW'S HIERARCHY

The five levels of basic needs proposed by Maslow's Hierarchy (Maslow, 1968) serve as a framework for the aspect of treatment the authors are proposing. In summary, Maslow's theoretical five-level hierarchy consists of physiological needs; safety needs; need for love, affection, and belonging; esteem; and self actualization. At the most basic level, physiological needs are the strongest and consist of necessities such as oxygen, food, and water. When physiological needs are satisfied and no longer paramount in an individual's thoughts and behaviors, the need for physical safety and security can become active. While adults who do not have this concern typically have little awareness of security needs, persons in developing areas where crime and theft are common constantly have this element of security instability. Under these conditions, it is challenging, and often inconceivable, for an individual to move beyond this immediate need, owing to often living in a state of "emergency." When the need for safety and physiological well-being are satisfied, the need for love, affection, and belongingness can emerge. When the first three levels of need are satisfied, the needs for self-esteem can become dominant. According to Maslow, humans have a need for a "stable, firmly based, high level of self-respect, and respect from others." It is not until this need is satisfied that a person feels self-confident and valuable in the world. When these needs are frustrated, the individual feels "inferior, weak, helpless and worthless." When all of the foregoing needs are satisfied, then and only then is the need for self-actualization, or "a person's need to be and do that which the person was 'born to do'" (Maslow, 1968).

A key aspect of Maslow's model is the hierarchical nature of the needs. The lower the needs in the hierarchy, the more fundamental they are and the more a person will tend to abandon higher needs in order to attempt to sufficiently meet lower needs (Maslow, 1943). This model raises both questions and possible answers concerning fundamental aspects of human nature and psychological well-being and what is needed to promote, maintain, and restore mental and emotional well-being (Maslow, 1968).

It appears that most traditional HIV treatment models address phys-iological aspects of care. However, the idea of promoting well-being goes beyond merely providing medications to those who are ill. Rather, it is a holistic concept that looks to assisting an individual to "thrive" and "restore mental and emotional well being," two ideas evident in Maslow's hierarchy.

One could surmise that many individuals living in developing coun-tries and facing poverty and disease-ridden circumstances are at the most basic level and are unable to thrive. It is hardly a stretch to recog-nize that the elimination of, or at minimum a decrease in, poverty as a stressor would lead to an increase in resiliency and a better chance of positive response and increased life span under ARV therapies. When one considers the global burden of poverty and treatment necessary to care for infected individuals, one quickly realizes that new systems must have measures for sustainability after global contributions are largely exhausted. Therein lies the case for including economic de-velopment considerations in the treatment of individuals infected with HIV/AIDS.

Education and Economic Development Linkage

It can be argued that the behavior of an individual at a particular moment is usually determined by his or her strongest need. This was evident in 1939 when Abraham Maslow initiated his investigations which culminated his five basic goals or "needs." These needs (physiological issues, safety, love, self-esteem, and self-actualization) are divided into two groupings: deficiency needs and growth needs. Within the deficiency needs, each lower need must be met before moving to the next higher level. Even once each of these needs has been satisfied, if at some future time a deficiency is detected, the individual is motivated to remove the deficiency. In the context of the current South African epidemiology, one should argue that the individual's need for basic nutrition and sustenance (deficiency need) will eclipse the need for health care (growth need) and ARVs. However, without the skill base to work or the access to gainful employment, there are no means to provide sustenance for themselves (with a benefit of increased self-worth and self-esteem) and their family. Thus, the basic demand for nourishment goes unaddressed. With nutritional and financial sustenance ameliorated, the concerns of health care and ARV adherence would become more able to be addressed.

Considering physiological intervention and Maslow's concepts, it appears evident that there is a need for nutrition and illness education intervention. For instance, the 1999 South African National Food Consumption Survey (Integrated Nutrition Programme, 1999) determined that malnutrition significantly impacts worker performance. The malnutrition-infection complex is well known in adult progression from HIV to AIDS, accompanying loss of productivity through the impact on adult physical performance and work capacity. Thus, if malnutrition issues are remedied, workers can return to their gainful employment or commence with entrepreneurial economic endeavors and become, or continue to become, productive members of society. Though in theory it seems like a simple solution, the loss of even a day's work for the very poor can be catastrophic in terms of the ability to feed their families. Often, these unfortunate circumstances will lead to an individual's sinking further into debt and spiraling into abject poverty or begging, resulting in absolute loss of self-worth and confidence. However, creating a small chance for economic revival will serve two purposes—the PLWHA will be able to take time to regenerate, become healthier, and let the treatment have a fuller effect and the opportunity to maintain or achieve even modest financial advantage is not eluded.

Economic Development Approaches

Presently, the UN Millennium Indicators report deterioration in most areas related to Millennium Development in South Africa (UN,

2005). There is little question that improvement must be made in each area to accomplish the desired goals by 2015. Each of the areas addressed within this proposed treatment framework directly support several the Millennium Development Goals (MDG). Specifically, MDG III, "Development and poverty eradication: The millennium development goals," focuses on sustainable development through poverty eradication with emphasis on decreasing the number of individuals who presently live on one dollar a day or less. The UN states very succinctly that "any effort to achieve sustainable development demands a concerted effort to reduce poverty, including finding solutions to hunger, malnutrition and disease (p. 2)." The progression toward an individual-based economic intervention opportunity to alleviate economic stress appears essential. Unfortunately, South African poverty statistics are startling, yet familiar, despite South Africa's being an upper-middle-income country. The country's distribution of wealth is among the most unequal in the world, with more than 19 million people living in the poorest 40% of households and earning below R360 (approximately $58 US) per adult per month. The majority of households either experience poverty or are particularly vulnerable to falling into poverty, with more than 10 million earning less than R192 (approximately $31 US) per adult per month. Many of these individuals are PLWHA, further compounding issues of stigma surrounding the illness and contributing to despair, depression, and suicide (Baingana, 2005).

The issue of sustainable development is one of psychological importance, as explained earlier in the context of Maslow's theory. There are two approaches to creating economic stability for a woman who is both stricken with poverty and enduring AIDS treatment. These two viable solutions are supportive employment and entrepreneurship. Supportive employment is defined as a work situation wherein the woman has a fixed work schedule and salary and is able to sustain the home and provide for her family, notwithstanding missing a day of work for treatment. It has been proven that work situations wherein a woman is worried about receiving treatment owing to potential loss of income can be detrimental to the effectiveness of the treatment and is counter-productive toward prolonging the progression of the illness. By creating a situation where the PLWHA is gainfully employed in a supportive environment, the effectiveness of the treatment and the mental well-being of the woman are both satisfactorily addressed.

Another way of operationalizing sustainable development could also take the form of microloans for use as a perpetual source of finance for entrepreneurial ventures as well as nutritional, educational, and food support. Perhaps a cliché, the phrase by Lao Tzu—"Give a man a fish and you feed him for a day. Teach him how to fish and you feed him for a lifetime"—has direct applicability. Microloans actually create opportunities for growth and mental balance. If a PLWHA is not an entrepreneur, the loan allows her to supply her family with better living conditions, food, and environment, therefore increasing the likelihood that she can retain a job and not struggle below the poverty line. In both cases, supported employment and individuals using microloans and microcredit are required to attend classes about finance, budgeting, and day-to-day expenses to help equip the individual with tools to provide for her family.

A number of documents (Daley-Harris, 2005; UN, 2006) clearly show microfinance as a viable poverty alleviation strategy at the local, national and global levels. Such a strategy also presents the perfect vehicle for offering health education to large groups of poor and very poor women. Health education leads to empowerment, which is directly involved in the increase of self-esteem and reaching self-actualization.

With the rapidly spreading AIDS pandemic, as well as other scourges of poverty such as tuberculosis and malaria, providing a comprehensive form of microenterprise that offers health education and health services is key in combating poverty and instability. Microenterprise programs provide a unique opportunity for reaching millions of clients, particularly poor women, with information and other kinds of support for HIV prevention and care. Linking client groups to HIV and other health information and services provides a new opportunity to massively increase AIDS prevention activities.

Microenterprise is a key, yet underutilized, mechanism for delivering on-the-ground solutions to mitigate the devastating impacts of HIV. One group (Nimatallah, 2006) indicates that "in Uganda, 75–80 percent of borrowers in Foundation for International Community Assistance (FINCA) programs are caring for AIDS orphans. A survey of 750 Opportunity International clients in Uganda and Zimbabwe revealed that, on average, these clients cared for 2.3 AIDS orphans each and that thirty percent of their business income is diverted to AIDS-related expenses." This example is indicative of a potential way that microenterprise could assist people out of poverty while providing education about protection against HIV/AIDS, TB, and malaria.

This author's proposed conceptual care idea does not stop at treating the patient's total body and immediate mental state but extends to include those factors that might impact the patient's state of mind and therefore affect the viability of the treatment. For instance, if a PLWHA is undergoing ARV therapy with some aspect of education about HIV/AIDS, yet this therapeutic regimen is without additional counseling education about managing said illness, with respect to family life and his or her everyday existence, then there is an entire facet of care being overlooked—the factoring of other stresses that the illness may add to the individual's life. However, a truly holistic approach, such as the one proposed by the authors, would address economic concerns and try to alleviate some of the psychosocial tensions the individual may be facing, which could undermine ARV treatment effectiveness.

Successes of the Microcredit Program

According to the State of Microcredit Campaign (Daley-Harris, 2005), of the 66.6 million poorest clients reached at the end of 2004, 83.5% (or 55.6 million) were women. The number of very poor women reached has grown from 10.3 million at the end of 1999 to 55.6 million at the end of 2004. This is a 440% increase from December 31, 1999, to December 31, 2004. This increase represents an additional 45.3 million of the poorest women receiving microloans in the last 5 years. Considering these statistics, one can see the significance microcredit has had for women across the world. This "reach" translates into success stories of women who have HIV, or are otherwise ill, in a multitude of ways. Microfinance institutions such as CRECER, Pro Mujer in Bolivia, and BRAC and Grameen Bank in Bangladesh are successfully integrating education with microfinance programming. The following are two examples of the positive impact of microcredit (Daley-Harris, 2005).

Case One. Susan W grew up in a poor, rural area of Kenya. She was forced to drop out of school after the fourth grade when her family could no longer afford the school fees and was thrown out of her house when she became pregnant at 17. Susan and her infant son moved to Nairobi, where she married and had a daughter. Her husband left her when they learned she was HIV-positive. Unable to find work and with no means to support her two small children, Susan ended up in prostitution. Susan learned about Jamii Bora, a Nairobi-based microfinance institution, from neighbors in her slum. She completed their business training, which gave her the skills and confidence to begin her clothes-mending and sales business. The microfinance services enabled her to quit prostitution and move her family from a shack in their crime- and disease-ridden slum into a safer house. Their house has a floor, running water, a waterproof roof, and locking door—

all luxuries they did not have previously. With each increasing loan, Susan buys more raw materials in bulk at lower costs, thus increasing her business's profitability. She is convinced she would not be alive without Jamii Bora's medical insurance and access to HIV medication, and can't imagine what would become of her children, as there is no one else to care for them. Susan has savings for the first time and is striving to earn enough to ensure her children's educations so they can break free from the chains of poverty.

Case Two. Janèt Dèval, a client of Fonkoze, a microcredit institution in Haiti, is one of the 66.6 million poorest clients reached. Janèt has been a credit client for more than 2 years and comes regularly to all meetings. She has also been a part of every literacy program available and is about to start the newest module on developing business skills. Not only could she not read or write when she started, but she has had an extra challenge: Janèt has only a fraction of her hearing due to an injury when she was 20 years old.

"My husband didn't want me to send my five children to school because his parents didn't send him to school. From the beginning, he said he would not pay and he has never given even one goud, but I always knew it was important. For a long time I have gone to Port-au-Prince to buy goods to sell in Hinche, and I put all my money into paying for school for my children. When I found out that Fonkoze gave literacy classes for market women, I was so happy. I never went to school even one day. I didn't know anything about school. I started right away with basic literacy and I have tried to never miss a class. I couldn't write my name and I didn't understand anything, but I kept going even when my husband got angry. My kids pushed me and encouraged me and they helped me practice my letters. The monitor, Christa, told me to keep writing every day even when I didn't understand. I can write my name now, and I write it everywhere. Imagine, I used to go to Port-au-Prince to buy and I couldn't read the bags and I felt lost. I couldn't keep track of what I bought. The drivers sometimes would take my boxes off the truck and give them to someone else, but I didn't know until I got all the way home. Now, I can't lose anything. Now I write my name on every box and I know what I buy. I finished Alfa Baz and Alfa Pos and then I went to the Health Program, too. I still don't know many things, so I want to keep going. I take my notebook to my school and I write in it because one day I hope to read and understand everything. I bought two books in the market and my kids help

me read them. I work hard in the market so that I can repay my
loans, keep going to school and so that my kids have that chance,
too. If my parents would have sent me to school, I would have
thrown a party for them to say thank you."

These success stories demonstrate the possibility of transferability
to other countries and regions of the world if developed and implemented in such a way that host countries could recognize there was an
ultimate impact to the country GDP. Not only do these stories illustrate
the success of the microloan program in general, they also reiterate
the demonstrable success that pairing HIV/AIDS treatments and continuing education classes have on the total picture. These women are
not only able to make their finances work; they are empowered and
strengthened by the program.

"Health Care Concept" Expansion

The connection between personal economic issues or "economic
development" and public health considerations in a "whole person"
treatment approach to HIV/AIDS has largely been absent or vaguely
alluded to in other academic papers and in some forums even rejected.
In a recent report the State of the Microcredit Summit Campaign (Da-
ley Harris, 2005) made a telling statement that speaks to this rejection:
"Those who say we cannot reach the very poor see no reason to try
and will, in fact, not reach the very poor. Those who say we cannot
integrate financial services with health education will see no reason
to try." This transition of thought proposed in this concept article
requires that components from a multitude of disciplines be married to
be truly effective. Thus, the proposed framework will require a shift in
thinking across disciplines of social work, psychology, public health,
and business, from acceptance of a silo structure toward embracing a
greater macrosystems change.

Expanding the concept idea of "health care" to address not only
the basic needs of a human, but to incorporate education, treatment,
and care of emotional and mental stress factors (i.e., supporting one's
family when one is afflicted with an illness) will improve treatment
response. The hopeful overall outcome is to bolster the infected population to be healthier and more responsive. In the language of Maslow,
with such a care approach, one can diminish the stress caused by the
lack of fulfillment of basic needs and transform a person into someone
capable of building on the satisfaction of their basic need to achieve
a higher social strata and economic success.

CONCLUSION

HIV/AIDS has changed from a "health issue to a development crisis" argues the Secretary-General of UNAIDS (UNAIDS 1999). Owing to this crisis, the ability of sub-Saharan African states to increase economic activity and social well-being is threatened. Economic development requires a strong working-age population for agriculture, education, industrial work, and other sectors of economic activity. This requires individuals to be strong both physiologically and psychologically, and to possess the necessary self-esteem to embark upon personal economic development efforts.

The approach described for holistic care of PLWHA is a unique solution not only to treating the physical illness itself but to increasing overall mental health, empowerment, and education for the PLWHA as well as her family unit. By approaching the illness as a total package rather than solely a physical manifestation of infirmity, the multi-faceted solution of economic development efforts and required courses and training solves these issues simultaneously. As the case studies have shown, not only are women in economically depressed countries and situations given tools to aid them in providing for their family, budgeting their time and money, and instilling them with a sense of accomplishment; these programs have also served to empower the women in their personal lives and achieve a stronger sense of self.

REFERENCES

Baingana, F., Thomas, R., & Comblain, C. (2005, January). *HIV/AIDS and mental health*. World Bank Human Development Network Discussion Paper (p. 11).
Daley-Harris, Sam. (2005). State of the Microcredit Summit Campaign Report 2005. Washington, D.C.: The Microcredit Summit Campaign.
De Cock, K. M., & Janssen, R. S. (2002). An unequal epidemic in an unequal world. *JAMA, 288,* 236–238.
Evans, S., Ferrando, S., et al. (1998). Pain and depression in HIV illness. *Psychosomatics, 39,* 528–535.
Gallego, L., Gordillo, V., & Catalan, J. (2000). Psychiatric and psychological disorders associated to HIV infection. *AIDS Reviews, 2*(1), 49–54.
Greenfield, S. F., Reizes, J. M., Magruder, K. M., Muenz, L. R., Kopans, B., & Jacobs, D. G. (1997). Effectiveness of community-based screening for depression. *American Journal of Psychiatry, 154,* 1391–1397.
Maslow, A. (1968). *Toward a psychology of being,* 2nd ed. New York: Van Nystrand.

Singh, N., Berman, S., Swindells, S., et al. (1999). Adherence of human immuno-deficiency virus-infected patients to antiretroviral therapy. *Clinics in Infectious Diseases, 29,* 824–830.

UNAIDS (2005) AIDS epidemic update. Geneva: Author.

UNAIDS/WHO (2004b). 2004 AIDS epidemic update. Geneva: Author.

United Nations Department of Economic Affairs and United Nations Capital Development Fund. Building Inclusive Financial Sectors for Development. United Nations, New York, 2006.

Uys, L. R. (2002). The practice of community caregivers in a home-based HIV/AIDS project in South Africa. *Journal of Clinical Nursing, 11*(1), 99–108.

Webb-Robins, L., Wilson, Z., & Flemengas, M. (2006, in press). Analysis of HIV caregivers in South Africa.

Wessels C., van Kradenburg J., Aronson W., Wilson Z., & Stein D. J. (1998). An "Anxiety Disorders Screening Day" in South Africa [letter]. *South African Medical Journal, 88:* 333–334.

World Bank. (2005). The World Bank's Global HIV/AIDS Program of Action. Washington, DC: Author.

World Health Organization. (2001). Macroeconomics and health: Investing in Health for economic development. Geneva: World Health Organization.

Gendered Economic, Social, and Cultural Challenges to HIV/AIDS Prevention and Intervention for Chinese Women

Catherine So-kum Tang

Asia and the Pacific are now the epicenter of the HIV/AIDS global pandemic, accounting for 24% of the world's new HIV infection and 21% of all people living with HIV/AIDS. In 2004, an estimated 8.2 million adults and children living in this region were infected with HIV, and about 540,000 people died of AIDS (Joint United Nations Program on HIV/AIDS [UNAIDS], 2005). In Asia, China is experiencing one of the most rapidly expanding HIV epidemics in the world. With over 1 billion people in China, even a relatively low HIV prevalence in the general population will translate into millions of infected cases. Similar to other countries, the percentage of women living with HIV/AIDS in China has also risen significantly (UNAIDS & WHO, 2004). Despite this alarming trend, the vulnerability of women being infected with HIV is much neglected in China. The current focus of HIV/AIDS and related prevention and intervention programs is mainly targeted at Chinese men (Center for Strategic and International Studies [CSIS], 2004). This article provides an analysis of gender-related economic, social, and cultural challenges to individual as well as nation-wide efforts in confronting the HIV/AIDS epidemic in Chinese women.

THE EVOLVING HIV/AIDS EPIDEMIC IN CHINA

The HIV/AIDS epidemic in China began in the early 1990s among needle-sharing, injecting drug users (IDUs) in the border provinces. The second epidemic was found among commercial blood donors, mostly poor farmers, and their families in the middle provinces. The current epidemic is related to China's rapid industrialization, urbanization, and economic reforms in recent years, with which there is increasing population mobility from rural villages to urban cities as well as an explosion of the commercial sex industry, especially in the eastern provinces. The rates of sexually transmitted infection (STI) have doubled since 1996, and the HIV/AIDS epidemic has begun to spread sexually from source populations to the general population. Among official documented cases of HIV/AIDS in China at the end of 2003 (Chinese Ministry of Health and UN Theme Group on HIV/AIDS in China [CMHUN], 2003), 51% contracted the disease as a result of injecting drugs, 21% as a result of un-hygienic blood plasma donations, 7.5% as a result of sexual trans-mission, and about 1% as a result of mother-to-child transmission (MTCT). China is currently experiencing a 30% annual rate of in-crease of reported HIV infection. With this rate of increase, there could be 10–20 million Chinese infected with HIV by 2010 (CMHUN, 2003).

Globally, the growing number of women infected with HIV is a dominant feature of the evolving epidemic (UNAIDS, UNFPA, & UNIFEM, 2004). Women now represent half of all adults living with HIV/AIDS, with the percentage as high as 60% among young women between the ages of 15 and 24. The rapid spread of the HIV/AIDS epidemic to women is also evident in China. During the period between 1990 and 2003, the male-to-female ratio in persons living with HIV/AIDS has narrowed dramatically from 9:1 to 4:1 in China and to 2:1 in Hong Kong. This translates into a nearly fourfold increase in prevalence among women in recent years, from approximately 0.008% in 1997 to 0.03% in 2003. The HIV prevalence rates of pregnant women also increased from 1% in 1996 to 3% in 2000. It was estimated that there were about 200,000–300,000 Chinese women of childbearing age living with HIV/AIDS in 2003 (UNAIDS & WHO, 2004).

Gender-Related HIV/AIDS Vulnerability in Chinese Women

There are differences between men and women in the natural course and prevention efforts of HIV/AIDS. Globally, women's risk of HIV infection from unprotected sex with infected men is much greater than the risk to men of having unprotected sex with infected women. Women as compared to men are exposed to the infection earlier, are often diagnosed later, and have higher mortality rates (UNAIDS et al., 2004). Women can also pass the infection to a baby during pregnancy, delivery, or breastfeeding. The primary method for preventing sexual transmission of the disease among sexually active individuals is male condom use, which is a male-controlled prevention measure. Female as compared to male condoms are more expensive as well as less available in most parts of the world. Given the foregoing gender differences, specific vulnerabilities and needs of women must be addressed in order to curtail the spread of the HIV/AIDS epidemic in Chinese women.

According to the gender and power theory (Connell, 1987; Wingood & DiClemente, 1996), women's risks of HIV infection is heavily influenced by socioeconomic factors, power imbalances within relationships, and gender-specific cultural norms. Indeed, rigid gender norms, widespread of gender-based violence (GBV), fear of men's violence, and poverty have been repeatedly cited as being instrumental to the "feminization" of the HIV/AIDS epidemic (UNAIDS et al., 2004; WHO, 2004). Thus, it is important to examine Chinese women's vulnerability to HIV/AIDS in light of a long history of patriarchy as well as rapid social and economic changes in China.

Gendered Cultural Vulnerability of Chinese Women

Gender scholars have argued that the global HIV/AIDS epidemic in women is largely related to women's inability to challenge male supremacy with their inherent inferior position in heterosexual sexual relationship, in the family, and in the society that makes women less able than men in exercising control over their bodies and lives (Connell, 1987; Wingood & DiClemente, 1996). In China, strong patriarchal influences still persist and remain salient, especially among older people and rural villagers. The latter two groups together comprise almost three-fourths of China's population. According to Chinese patriarchy, men are expected to have multiple sex partners, while premarital chastity and marital fidelity are emphasized in women. Men are often in control of both sexual and reproductive decision making, such as when and how a woman will have sexual relations. Gendered division of labor between "reproductive" roles for women and "productive" roles for men has limited Chinese women's access to the paid labor market. This reinforces Chinese women's social and economic dependence on men and compels the former to have early marriages, tolerate sexual behaviors imposed by their male partners, and engage in sex trade. Sexual violence against Chinese women by men in the form of date rape, marital rape, or child sexual abuse predisposes women to high risks of STI and HIV/AIDS. Social stigma and fear of violence also prevent many Chinese women from accessing HIV/AIDS information, from asking their male sexual partner to wear condoms, from getting diagnostic tests, and from seeking treatment for the infection. Even the act of carrying condoms has different symbolic meanings for Chinese men and women. Having condoms available for use represents sexual vigor and potency for Chinese men but may serve as a "proof" of prostitution or promiscuity for Chinese women (Fung & Chung, 1999; Tang, Wong, & Lee, 2001).

Another powerful cultural influence in Chinese societies is the Confucian doctrines that emphasize familism, harmony, and social order. These doctrines prescribe a hierarchy of social relationships with clear roles and duties. The Confucian concept of model womanhood commands the submission of Chinese wives to their husbands, and this still persists as the protocol for proper family life in China. Marital roles of Chinese couples are gender-segregated according to their traditional gender roles, and husbands often dominate over major decision making in various family matters (Choi & Lee, 1997; Tang, 1999). Chinese men as heads of households are socialized to believe they are entitled to use violence in the family to assert their own dominant status to maintain order in the family. Many Chinese women still consider they should be sexually available to their husbands and see this as an intrinsic part of the role of being a "good" wife, even though this may conflict with their own sexual desires and the need to protect themselves from STI or HIV. In a large community survey in Hong Kong, 15% of the surveyed Chinese women felt satisfying their husband's sexual needs were more important than adopting safer sex practices, about 7% said their husband insisted on condom-less sexual intercourse, and 2% were afraid that their husband might become violent if the latter was asked to wear condoms (Tang et al., 2001). Thus, it is not surprising that condom use rate is low (about 30%) among Chinese couples.

Gendered Social-Economic Vulnerability of Chinese Women

China has been experiencing rapid economic and social changes in recent years. This has led to population shift from rural villages to urban cities, explosion of the commercial sex trade, disruptions of social systems, and widespread GBV. With their inherent inferior social status and economic disadvantage, Chinese women are particularly vulnerable to adverse consequences of these social changes.

Low Level of Awareness of HIV/AIDS. Sex is still a taboo topic in China, and open discussion about sexual matters is uncommon among Chinese (Fung & Chung, 1999; Zhang, Li, Li, & Beck, 1999). Moreover, China has had a national "one-child" population policy for several decades. Effective contraception has become the top priority in Chinese couples' sexual life. The general community has learned to associate condoms as a contraceptive device rather than as an effective means of disease control. Thus, there is a general low level of awareness of HIV/AIDS and its prevention. For example, in a survey of community adults in China conducted in 2002 (Futures Group, 2002), more than three-fourths of city residents (men and women) did not feel personally at risk of HIV infection, and only 3% spontaneously connected condom use with precautions against STI and HIV.

Disparities in HIV/AIDS awareness exist among people with different sociocultural backgrounds. Rural villagers as compared to urban dwellers, older as compared to younger people, and women as compared to men are less likely to have heard of HIV/AIDS and to know about the role condoms can play in reducing the spread of HIV (Futures Group, 2002). The lack of awareness of the HIV/AIDS epidemic and its prevention could be related to Chinese women's low level of education. In China, the current adult illiteracy rates are 22% for women as compared to only 8% for men. Under the patriarchal traditions in China, girls and women are often disadvantaged in receiving even basic education. Girls are less likely than boys to attend school because parents are more likely to spend resources on educating sons than on daughters. Many families do not understand the benefits of educating girls, whose role is often narrowly viewed as being prepared for marriages, motherhood, and domestic responsibilities. Young women are often placed with a high burden of domestic tasks, childcare responsibilities, and caregiving obligations for elder and sick family members. They are thus relatively house-bound and have limited time to acquire new knowledge and skills. They generally have a level of awareness of their own vulnerability to the HIV/AIDS epidemic.

Population Mobility and Migrant Workers. As economic development accelerates in China, there is massive rural-to-urban migration. More than 120 million Chinese have temporarily relocated from poor rural areas to cities or towns in search of work, and are often referred to as the "floating population." These migrant workers are mostly men, young, unmarried, and with limited education. They have left its original place of residence, customs, and norm and face enormous changes and pressures in morality, life style, scope of contact, and sexual behavior. With increased freedom but general ignorance, many economic migrants may find themselves engage in illicit activities and risky sexual behavior (Tucker et al., 2005). The practice of unprotected sex is common in migrant workers, with 30% indicating never using a condom in their sexual encounters (Ma et al., 2002).Young female migrant workers are also subject to a high risk of coercive sexuality by their coworkers and employers. A recent study has found that 1.4% of migrant workers were HIV-positive, a much higher prevalence than that found in the general population in China.

Migrant workers are generally unwilling to seek testing or treatment for STI or HIV in hospitals or clinics, owing to fear of discrimination (such as losing their employment) and the high cost of medical care. They thus create a large bridging population from high- to low-risk individuals (Tucker et al., 2005), especially to women in rural communities. With increased income, unmarried male migrant workers are now more able to find a wife in the villages to start their families. These married migrant workers will need to travel frequently from cities to their rural homes for family reunion. This will bring an unknown risk of sexual transmission of HIV to their rural wives, who are already reporting high rates (60%) of gynecological infections (Kaufman & Jing, 2002). Owing to high service charges, long distances from clinics, and a shortage of doctors, most rural women do not receive prompt and quality testing and treatment of STI and HIV. They also suffer from high risks of iatrogenic infection, owing to poor sanitation in remote rural areas, shortage of proper equipment, ineffective sterilization of medical equipment, and lack of training in universal precautions. This will result in late diagnosis and high mortality of HIV/AIDS and related infection in rural women.

Commercial Sex Trade. There is increasing commercial sex trade in China in recent years, especially in the eastern provinces. It is estimated that about 17–40% of men had engaged in commercial sex in China (Lau & Siah, 2001; Ma et al., 2002; Pan, 2001). Most of them are married, middle-class, and younger than 35 years. With rapid economic reforms and growth in the country, there are increasing opportunities to obtain extra disposable income to purchase sex among the newly wealthy businessmen and young migrant workers. Commercial sex clients often engage in high-risk sexual behavior, which is an important mode of HIV transmission. Lau and Siah (2001) found that 27% of commercial sex clients did not always use condoms and 1–4% had practiced unprotected anal intercourse with commercial sex workers. And about 1.5% of commercial sex clients contracted STI and HIV as a result of sexual contacts with female sex workers (FSWs). Unfortunately, 38% of commercial male sex clients also failed to use condoms with their regular female marital partners, thus exposing a sizable number of women to unknown risk of STI and HIV infection.

It is estimated that there are more than 3 million sex workers in China, mostly women. There are at least 12 distinct types of sex workers, ranging from courtesans or escorts to brothel-based sex workers to freelance street walkers, with a diversity of work organizations, income, clientele, and employment status. Most FSWs came from remote rural areas, are poorly educated, and have little knowledge about HIV. For example, about 14–30% of surveyed FSWs knew that a condom would prevent HIV infection, but only 2–30% considered themselves at risk for HIV infection. Also, FSWs are the least able and likely to negotiate protected sex with their clients, because of their low social status. About 40% of FSWs reported having engaged in condom-less sexual activities with their clients (UNAIDS & WHO, 2004). Thus, prevalence rates of STIs (22–73%) and HIV infections (15–18%) in FSWs are much higher than the general population. The most vulnerable sex workers are women and girls illegally trafficked across borders for the sex trade, who are most likely to become infected during the first 6 months of their stay. Very often, they need to continue to have unprotected sex even after discovering symptoms of a STI in themselves or in their clients. There is also a relatively small number of male sex workers who would serve both male and female clients. High-risk sexual behavior is also noted among men who had sex with men, with 30% having multiple partners, 37% engaging in anal sex, and 40–67% reporting inconsistent condom uses (Lau, Siah, & Tsui, 2002).

Gender-based Violence. GBV is now the leading factors for HIV/ AIDS epidemic in women across countries (UNAIDS et al., 2004). Women who are beaten or emotionally dominated by their partners are much more likely to become infected by HIV (Martin & Curtis, 2004). Women who experience forced sex not only are unable to negotiate condom use but related abrasions and cuts would also facilitate the entry of HIV when it is present. Being a victim of sexual violence will also increase the likelihood of engaging in subsequent unprotected sex, having multiple partners, participating in sex work, and substance use, which are risk factors for HIV infection (UNAIDS et al., 2004; WHO, 2002).

There is limited information on sexual coercion among Chinese women, given the immense stigma attached to sexual victimization. In Hong Kong, 3–7% of the surveyed community women reported being sexually coerced by their spouses (Hong Kong Social Welfare Dept, 2005), and 7–36% of surveyed adolescent girls were forced to have sex with either peers or adults (Tang, 2006). However, it should be noted that GBV has been a problem in Chinese societies for many centuries, given Chinese culture embraces rigid gender norms and emphasizes patriarchy values, familism, and social order that are conducive to the exploitation of women (Tang, Wong, & Cheung, 2002). Chinese women are typically charged with the responsibility of maintaining family integrity and ensuring social stability. Policies designed to keep the family intact also function to keep a significant proportion of women exposed to unknown risks for intimate partner abuse and marital rape. For example, child sexual abuse and incest may be condoned as legitimate treatment of girls, as filial daughters should defer to their fathers, and marital rape or physical abuse is an acceptable means to discipline women when they are perceived as failing to meet the prescribed cultural and social standard of obedient wives. Even nowadays, a woman who survived acquaintance rape is still expected to marry her rapist to preserve her chastity and to avoid social disgrace to her family.

Stigma and Discrimination. In China, there is widespread stigma and discrimination toward people living with HIV/AIDS. For example, fewer than half of respondents to a survey thought that HIV-infected people should be allowed to return to work, and many held that the HIV status about family members should be kept secret. Only one-third of respondents were willing to take care of a family member with HIV/AIDS (Futures Group, 2002). Other social surveys in China also showed that 60–75% of respondents said they would try to avoid contact with people living with HIV/AIDS, 45% believed HIV/AIDS was the result of low morals or punishment by God, 30% thought that these people should be cared for in a closed sanatorium, and about half of the surveyed health care workers preferred not to treat HIV/AIDS patients (Wang, 2000). These intolerant attitudes and discriminatory behaviors would severely impede prevention and intervention efforts against HIV/AIDS. People will again shun HIV/AIDS testing and treatment for fear of bringing stigma and shame to their families and losing their jobs. Chinese women are generally reluctant to sero-test for HIV (Ho & Loke, 2003), fearing that if they are tested positive, they would be divorced by their husband, evicted from their home, forced into sex work, and consequently be at risk for further discrimination and violence.

Challenges to HIV/AIDS Prevention and Intervention in China

The United Nations has urged a scaled-up response to curtail the rapid spread of the HIV/AIDS epidemic in China and Asia (UNAIDS, 2005). It is argued that evidence-based prevention measures, together with targeted care and treatment initiatives for people living with HIV, can reduce growth of the epidemic and its impact on individuals and communities. It is estimated that when simultaneously bringing prevention and treatment to scale, the Asia-Pacific region can cut the annual AIDS death rate in 2010 by nearly 40%, and the total HIV prevalence can also be reduced by more than 40% (UNAIDS, 2005). Currently, a number of prevention and intervention strategies have been initiated in China. The following analysis would highlight specific needs and concerns of Chinese women in order to further the effectiveness of these strategies.

HIV/AIDS Prevention and Control in China

The SARS crisis in China in early 2003 alerted the Chinese government to reexamine how her public health systems are structured to address challenges of infectious diseases such as HIV/AIDS. Since then, China has crafted national strategic treatment and care plans to indicate her "five commitments" in providing "four frees and one care" programs to fight against the HIV/AIDS epidemic: free antiretroviral drug treatment for poor citizens, free testing and counseling for poor citizens, free treatment to prevent mother-to-child transmission of HIV, free schooling for AIDS orphans, and care for families affected by HIV/AIDS. Senior government leaders have also committed to implementing harm-reduction strategies, including needle exchange and methadone substitution therapy for IUDs. Other programs such as 100% condom use, peer education, and public health outreach for commercial sex workers have also been piloted in some provinces. Legal reforms are currently underway to safeguard rights and confidentiality of infected individuals. However, there is not yet any national policy or plans to address the evolving HIV/AIDS epidemic in Chinese women, despite international organizations have called for concerted efforts to confront this pandemic health crisis in women (UNAIDS et al., 2004).

Prevention Strategies for Chinese Women

In order to target HIV/AIDS prevention programs for Chinese women, their specific needs and realities imposed by gender-related economic, social, and cultural obstacles must be addressed and tackled. These prevention approaches should be multifaceted, including strategies that fight against poverty, improve education, enhance HIV/AIDS awareness, facilitate the acquisition of new life-skills and behavior change, make available woman-centered health services, and bring an end to discrimination and GBV.

Eliminating Illiteracy and Improving Educational Opportunities. Education has an important impact on women's risk of contracting HIV (UNAIDS et al., 2004). This is of particular relevance to Chinese women given their high adult illiteracy rate and limited opportunities to acquire new information and knowledge. Education can affect HIV/AIDS prevalence rates and change Chinese women's lives by enhancing employment opportunities, facilitating economic independency, and reducing poverty. It can also increase Chinese women's self-confidence and decision-making power in the family and in the wider community, thus enabling them to take better control of their bodies and protect themselves from GBV. To be more effective in reducing the impact of HIV/AIDS, education curricula and systems in China should also be revisited to include mandates that not only impart pure knowledge but challenge and dispel long-rooted cultural gender stereotypes and misinformation. This entails not only increasing Chinese girls' access to schooling; free education and incentives should be offered to families to make it financially feasible for them to send their daughters to schools, especially in impoverished, remote, or rural areas. There should also be ongoing national efforts toward universal education for all Chinese girls and women.

Enhancing Knowledge about HIV/AIDS, Safer Sex, and Sexual Health. Many Chinese girls and women, especially illiterate or semi-illiterate women, know very little about their bodies, their sexual and reproductive health, or HIV/AIDS (Vandermoortele & Delamonica, 2000; UNAIDS, 2001). As open and direct sexual communication is uncommon in Chinese societies, Chinese women have limited channels and resources to acquire sex-related information. In China, there are about 100 million Chinese girls aged 15–24 who are about to embark on their sexual lives. They often receive little sex education beyond abstinence promotion in schools and have limited access to reproductive health counseling and services. Chinese married women also know very little about their personal vulnerability to HIV infection. A majority of them have little concern about contracting the disease from their husbands and believe there is no need for safer sex behaviors as along as they have sex with their husbands only (Tang et al., 2001). Thus, information about HIV/AIDS and the promotion of safer sex behaviors as well as sexual and reproductive health are at the core of prevention programs for Chinese women.

Accessing Condoms and Alternate Safer Sex Measures. Male and female condoms are the only technology that can prevent sexual transmission of HIV and other STI. Female condoms are still unavailable in many parts of China and cost much more than male condoms. As condom use typically represents sexual promiscuity and unfaithfulness of Chinese women, purchasing and possessing condoms may bring immense embarrassment, social disapproval, and stigma to Chinese women. Thus, condom promotion and distribution to Chinese women is often met with resistance from both men and women. In some provinces, local health regulation even prohibits the prescription or sale of condoms in public clinics and hospitals. Furthermore, health care providers may not counsel their woman patients about condom use as an effective measure against HIV/AIDS beyond contraception. Thus, effective HIV/AIDS prevention programs should promote positive social attitudes toward condom. Information about condoms and their use should be provided to Chinese women to dispel myths and to reduce shame and embarrassment. Efforts should be made to ensure Chinese women have consistent access to high quality condoms, and less expensive female condoms should be made available so that Chinese women will have more control and initiation in HIV/AIDS prevention. Free distribution of condoms to high-risk groups such as FSWs may enhance their use, and subsequently reduce rates of HIV infection. Finally, Stein (1990) has argued that for empowering women against HIV infection, it is not by training them to be more assertive with male partners but by giving them tools to protect themselves such as vaginal virucide or microbicide. Thus, there is a need to also identify and develop alternate safer sex measures for Chinese women in addition to male and female condoms.

Empowering and Training for Life-Skills. For many Chinese women, knowledge and positive attitudes about safer sex practices is not enough. In fact, the ABCs—Abstain, Be faithful, and use Condoms—may not meet specific needs of some Chinese women given their inherent social inferiority and low economic status in the family and in the community (Martin & Curtis, 2004). For example, abstinence is meaningless to economically disadvantaged women who need to engage in CSW to earn a living. Faithfulness offers little protection to rural wives of migrant workers who may have several sex partners in their urban workplace or were already infected before they were married. Given unequal power within marital relationship, it is difficult for Chinese women to gain the cooperation of their dominant husbands to use condoms without threat or acts of violence, rejection, or abandonment. Chinese women need to learn not only how HIV is transmitted but how to negotiate safer sex relations given their specific gendered obstacles. In this regard, HIV/AIDS prevention programs should also address how Chinese women find safe ways to financially support themselves, to deal with intimae partner violence, to protect their reproductive and sexual health, and to learn to assert their human rights. Life-skills training in the form of personal empowerment lessons on assertiveness, communications, and negotiation is thus important for Chinese women. However, women's relationship patterns should also be taken into consideration when planning life-skills training programs for HIV/AIDS prevention. For example, younger women who are in unstable relationships with men tend to reject HIV health messages, and women who are in the process of arranging or stabilizing a sexual relationship are often reluctant to try out new life-skills (Barker, Battle, Cummings, & Bancroft, 1998). Legal and policy frameworks also need to be strengthened to support women's rights to economic independence by having the right to own and inherit land and property, by providing vocational training, and by prohibiting gender discrimination at work.

Making Women-Centered Health Services Available. Globally, only one-fifth of those who need HIV/AIDS prevention health services have access to them. Many individuals in poor and remote areas of developing countries have little or no access to these services. In China, HIV/AIDS prevention health services are still developing and are mainly found in large urban cities or in locations with a concentration of high-risk populations such as IDUs and FSWs. There is a great need to establish centers with comprehensive health services that focus on addressing women's special needs and barriers to HIV/AIDS prevention and sexual health. These centers should not only serve high-risk groups but target young girls and adult women in the mainstream. In addition to imparting sexual and safer sex education, these centers can also provide voluntary counseling and testing (VCT) for HIV and STI. VCT not only enables early detection of these diseases but can contribute to decreases in unprotected sexual relations, number of sexual partners, stigma associated with HIV/AIDS, and prevalence of mother-to-infant transmission of HIV and increases in condom use, abstinence, and utilization of other health services (UNAIDS et al., 2004). To encourage Chinese women to utilize these services when available, efforts should be made to reduce stigma and discrimination by ensuring confidentiality or by eliminating service fees for poor women. When financial and practical resources do not permit the establishment of these centers, existing health care facilities for women, including reproductive health centers and antenatal clinics, can be strengthened. Health service workers should also be prepared for the HIV epidemic in Chinese women and must learn basic prevention protocols for detection of STI and HIV/AIDS, opportunistic infections associated with HIV/AIDS, and MTCT of HIV.

Stopping Gender-Based Violence. GBV enforces Chinese women's subordination, endangers their physical and sexual health with increased vulnerability to HIV/AIDS and STI, prevents them from exercising their basic rights, and constrains their development. Community-wide public education is thus necessary to promote zero tolerance of GBV in marital/sexual relationship, in the family, and in the community and acknowledging that intimate partner violence, coercive sex, and gender inequity exacerbate the spread of HIV/AIDS. Rigid gender norms and commonly held gender myths should be challenged and dispelled. Of importance is that the underlying societal structures in China need to be reviewed and reformed to eliminate inherent differential power distribution between the two genders. Support for Chinese women who are victims of GBV is crucial, and rape/sexual violence clinics may be added to HIV/AIDS prevention service centers or vice versa. Legal reforms in terms of promoting Chinese women's legal rights, criminalization of rape and intimate partner violence, and early reporting and intervention of incidents of GBV can also facilitate the prevention of HIV and STI. Health care facilities in China can also be expanded to serve as a major entry point for ending violence, and health care workers need to be trained to recognize signs of GBV as well as to provide VCT for HIV and STIs. It is important to also involve Chinese men in anti-GBV campaigns in order to examine their own patriarchal attitudes and behaviors and to act as peer leaders. Chinese men can be partners with Chinese women to tackle the widespread of GBV in China. Men's fears and resistance in challenging the status quo of the two genders should be addressed. Workplace and school-based prevention education programs for boys and men about sexual violence can be implemented to address the interrelated problems of gender inequity, GBV, and HIV/AIDS. Training health care providers, teachers, and others will enable them to identify, counsel, and refer women victims of sexual violence to health services.

Intervention Strategies for Chinese Women

Of the 1 million people receiving HIV/AIDS treatment worldwide, the overwhelming majority are educated men living in urban areas in wealthy countries, where health services are generally better and more available than in rural areas in developing countries (UNAIDS & WHO, 2004). Women in developing countries, in particular, are underserved (UNAIDS et al., WHO). In China, 100,000 adults are in need of HIV/AIDS treatment, and the majority of service recipients are urban men. Gendered obstacles that hinder women's access to HIV/AIDS treatment are also evident in China. Many women are reluctant to receive treatment even when available because related programs are not developed with their special needs in mind. For example, without childcare or homecare support services, it is difficult for women to leave their children and families to attend treatment programs.

Wingood & DiClemente (1996) have noted that effective HIV/AIDS interventions for women tend to share several characteristics. They are guided by social psychological theory, include skills training in condom use and sexual communication, and emphasize gendered power imbalance and sexual assertiveness. They tend to be multiple-session programs that are strongly peer influenced through interaction and discussion, as well as being led by gender-sensitive health educators from similar ethnic, cultural, and marital background. Intervention of HIV/AIDS typically focuses on VCT, antiretroviral therapy (ART), and harm-reduction among high risk groups.

Voluntary Counseling and Testing

Goals of VCT in terms of treatment is to ensure those who are tested positive receive counseling about stigma and the impact of HIV as well as about ART. There are many barriers to sero-testing and subsequent treatment for Chinese women. In China, a majority of doctors are men with little training in HIV/AIDS, and they often endorse patriarchal beliefs about women. They generally lack awareness and sensitivity to women's vulnerability to HIV infection and may simply fail to refer women for testing and treatment in spite of relevant symptoms. Chinese women may fear disclosing serostatus to doctors for treatment owing to concerns about negative consequences with respect to jobs, marital relationship, and other aspects of life. Where VCT is available in the health care setting, Chinese women should also be encouraged to discuss their fear of violence if they disclose a positive status and receive referral for help as soon as possible. Adolescent girls particularly need confidentiality in counseling and care. Personnel working in these VCT centers should be sensitive to specific needs and concerns of women. For example, reproductive choices of pregnant women before VCT should be carefully discussed. Economic and cultural reasons for childbearing should be taken into consideration when a decision has to be made about delayed childbearing or termination of pregnancy if the sero-testing is positive. Sometimes, even if HIV-infected woman desires an abortion, she may not be able to get one; either her family cannot afford it or there is no safe facility in her area. Thus, VCT services should be in close partnership with relevant health care facilities and medical personnel such as obstetricians, gynecologists, and family planning doctors.

Antiretroviral Therapy

Similar to other countries, only a small proportion of HIV-infected Chinese men and women receive ART. Chinese women are not always able to use available HIV/AIDS treatment services because of their inferior status in the family and in the community. Where money is limited, families and societies often choose to pay for medications or treatments for men rather then for women. There are also more women than men lacking the money to pay for medications, treatment services, and transportation to treatment centers. In most parts of China, when pregnant women are tested HIV-positive, usually only a single dose of ART medication at the onset of labor is given to protect the infant during delivery. Very often, the infected women are left without ART after childbirth, especially if they are not breastfeeding. Thus, there is an urgent need to establish ART programs for infected Chinese women, and continuous treatment should be ensured for both infected mothers and their newborns. Attention should also be given to enhance drug adherence, given the many side effects of ART. Researchers have found that complex drug regiment did not compromise adherence in HIV-infected Chinese patients (Fong et al., 2003). Instead, poor adherence was linked to negative impacts on quality of life from drug side effects. Thus, drug treatment of HIV/AIDS can be enhanced by preparing Chinese women for potential side effects of their ART and managing the toxicity when present.

Combined Prevention and Intervention for FSW

The major source populations of sexual transmission for HIV in China are FSWs and their clients. Very often, only FSWs are targeted for HIV prevention and control, and their fundamental human rights issues are sometimes at stake. It is because the threat to public health typically takes over basic rights of these already marginalized women. China has had mandatory sex worker reeducation centers where FSWs are detained by police, tested without consent for HIV and other STIs, and then released. Reforms within these centers could provide an entry point for delivering HIV/AIDS prevention and intervention programs to FSWs, with close collaboration among public security bureau, police, and relevant health care services (Tucker et al., 2005). When FSWs are detained in these reformed reeducation centers, they can be provided with information about their personal vulnerability to HIV and STIs, education about prevention and treatment strategies for these diseases, and STI/HIV surveillance testing with informed consents. However, compulsory detention in reeducation centers and police crackdowns may also promote FSW mobility. This will increase these women's risk of STIs and distances them from regular health care and support network. When FSWs are driven underground, proper treatment of STIs and HIV is even more difficult.

FSWs frequently lack the negotiating experience and social capital to refuse unprotected commercial sex. Thus, involving their clients in STI and HIV prevention and intervention is equally important. HIV prevention efforts should also be directed at brothel owners and intermediaries. Peer support among FSWs is also important. Furthermore, identifying and improving sexual health of migrant men should also become a national priority for public health infrastructure in China. Indeed, pilot projects that have a focus on HIV/AIDS prevention and intervention in FSWs and their clients have shown promising results, with increases in knowledge about HIV transmission, more consistent condom use, and decreases in STI incidents among FSWs (Ma et al., 2002; UNAIDS & WHO, 2004).

Psychosocial Support

Globally, women who are diagnosed with AIDS survived for less time than men diagnosed with AIDS (UNAIDS et al., 2004). This greater mortality of women has been attributed to delayed diagnosis and less access to health care than for men. Another plausible explanation is that many of these women often lack social support and financial, medical, and legal resources to deal effectively with the disease. Having been infected with HIV is particularly difficult for Chinese women who are socialized with Confucian emphasis on women's reproductive and caregiver roles in the family. These women typically experience rejection and isolation by others, especially by unsupportive marital/sex partners, family members, and friends. They often feel stigmatization and shame owing to their illness, have great concerns about transmitting HIV to other family members, and are still expected to be caretakers of others even though they are sick themselves. When they are sick, there is often no one to provide care for them. They have immense anticipatory grief about losing their children, marital/sex partner, and existing social support, in addition to losing their own enjoyment of life and mortality. Many of them also experience psychological symptoms such as anxiety, depression, anger, insomnia, and memory loss. Thus, psychological intervention, including individual, marital, or group counseling, is also necessary for these women. It will enable them to verbalize their concerns, to ameliorate mental distress, to develop alternate coping strategies, and to gain support and cooperation of their spouse, family members, or friends during the course of treatment.

FUTURE DIRECTIONS

In recent years, the Chinese government has actively engaged in confronting the HIV/AIDS threat in China. National plans and policies have been crafted to tackle the epidemic. Similar to other developing countries in the Asia-Pacific region, China has yet to face critical challenges in HIV/AIDS prevention and control in coming years (UNAIDS, 2005). In spite of recent efforts such as the "five commitments" to provide "four frees and one care" programs; standardized training, treatment, and HIV/AIDS counseling are still under- or undeveloped in impoverished or rural regions of China. In general, very few programs have been rigorously evaluated for their effectiveness. Funding is insufficient, the health care infrastructure remains weak, and there is no national agency with authority to enforce recommendations. Nation-wide mechanisms to redress or prohibit discrimination against people living with HIV/AIDS are still developing. Most important of all, there is a lack of awareness and initiatives in addressing the evolving HIV/AIDS epidemic in Chinese women. There is an urgent need to expand the pool of gender experts in China to conduct a thorough gender analysis and design a national response to meet specific needs of men and women in combating the HIV/AIDS epidemic in China.

Strengthening HIV Testing and Surveillance Systems

The current HIV testing and surveillance system is mainly maintained by the Chinese Ministry of Health and Chinese Center for Disease Control. It has a short history and needs time and resources to strengthen its ability to compile, track, and monitor the totality of the HIV response programs in China. Currently, national guidelines and technical protocols for surveillance are not well defined, communicated, or universally followed. It is pointed out that the current testing and surveillance system represents only 3.7–7.4% of the total estimated HIV-positive population in China (CSIS, 2004). This means that only a small number of infected persons in China are aware of their status and known to the health care systems. The magnitude and trajectory of the evolving epidemic thus remains unclear, making prevention and targeted interventions a particular challenge. Furthermore, few reported statistics provided gender breakdowns, and important information about women is not available. Thus, this system needs further refinement and precision with gender segregation. Statistics should be reported separately for men and women so that specific rates and trends pertaining to Chinese women are available for comparison with Chinese men or women in other countries.

Ensuring Effective Diagnosis and Treatment

Given gender differences in the natural course and mortality of HIV/AIDS, efforts should be directed at addressing the serious lack of qualified personnel and the necessary equipment and technologies to properly diagnosis, counsel, treat, monitor, and care for women infected with HIV, especially for women residing in rural China. It is also important to ensure that woman patients are not just receiving treatment but can expect effective and gender-sensitive treatment, counseling, and follow-on care. Required drugs and tests should be made available at reasonable prices, and a national plan should be developed for access to treatment and care for all HIV-infected individuals in China, including women.

Establishing a Nation-Wide Public Health Infrastructure

According to WHO (2002), public health infrastructure is vital in order to define the magnitude, scope, characteristics, and consequences of various health issues, including HIV/AIDS; to identify vulnerability and protective factors that increase or decrease their prevalence; to determine salient components of prevention and intervention strategies; and to implement these programs in a variety of settings with continuous evaluation of their impact and cost-effectiveness (WHO, 2002). In China, pubic health infrastructure remains undeveloped in most rural areas. Hence, China's responses, such as prevention, harm reduction, and treatment programs, to health threats and epidemics have been severely undermined, as a large proportion of the population cannot be reached. To confront the HIV/AIDS crisis in China and its rapid spread to Chinese women, national efforts should be directed at establishing public health systems in remote and rural areas in addition to those in urban cities. These systems should not only note gender differences in the natural course of HIV/AIDS, but must address social, economic, and cultural obstacles that are specific to women in its prevention and treatment.

Mainstreaming Gender and Enhancing Civil and International Participation

Similar to women across countries, Chinese women's risk of HIV infection is amplified by gender-related socioeconomic factors, power imbalances between relationships, and patriarchal cultural norms (Connell, 1987; Wingood & DiClemente, 1996). In addressing the inequality between men and women in the sharing of power and decision-making at all levels, the Chinese government and her partners should devise an active and visible policy of mainstreaming gender perspectives in policy design and programs before decisions are taken. In confronting the HIV/AIDS epidemic in Chinese women, national polices should mandate new and existing funding be channeled to institute population-wide gender-sensitive prevention programs and to ensure equitable access to treatment and resources for men and women. Gender budgeting exercises are necessary to ensure budgetary allocations match with policy commitment, and resources are indeed utilized for the benefit of addressing women's specific needs in HIV/AIDS prevention and intervention. Currently, the Chinese government remains the major policy and program source. Concerted efforts could be made with local women's organizations as well as international women network to compile relevant information and to share realistic strategies that address the triple challenges of poverty, gender inequality, and HIV/AIDS in women across countries.

REFERENCES

Barker, J. C., Battle, R. S., Cummings, G. L., & Bancroft, K. N. (1998). Condoms and consequences: HIV/AIDS education and African American women. *Human Organization, 57,* 273–283.

Center for Strategic and International Studies. (2004). *Defusing China's time bomb: Sustaining the momentum of China's HIV/AIDS Response.* Washington, DC: Author.

Chinese Ministry of Health and UN Theme Group on HIV/AIDS in China. (2003). *A joint assessment of HIV/AIDS prevention, treatment and care in China.* Geneva: Author.

Choi, P., & Lee, C. (1997). The hidden abode of domestic labor: The case of Hong Kong. In F. Cheung (Ed.), *Engendering Hong Kong societies: A gender perspective of women's status,* (pp. 157–200). Hong Kong: The Chinese University Press.

Connell, R. W. (1987). *Gender and power.* Stanford, CA: Stanford University Press.

Fong, O., Ho, C., Fung, L., Lee, F., Tse, W., Yuen, C., et al. (2003). Determinants of adherence to highly active antiretroviral therapy (HAART) in Chinese HIV/AIDS patients. *HIV Medicine, 4,* 133–138.

Fung, E., & Chung, S. (1999). *Survey on women & AIDS.* Hong Kong: St. John's Cathedral HIV Information and Drop-in Center.

Futures Group—China. (2002). *Attitudes towards HIV/AIDS in China: Research on public knowledge, attitudes and behaviour in cities and towns.* China: Author.

Ho, C., & Loke, A. (2003). Pregnant women's decisions on antenatal HIV screening in Hong Kong. *AIDS Care, 15,* 821–827.

Hong Kong Social Welfare Department. (2005). *Study on child abuse and spouse battering.* Hong Kong: Author.

Joint United Nations Program on HIV/AIDS (UNAIDS). (2001). *HIV/AIDS: China's titanic peril, 2001 Update of the AIDS situation and needs assessment report.* Geneva: Author.

Joint United Nations Program on HIV/AIDS (UNAIDS). (2005). *A scaled-up response to AIDS in Asia and the Pacific.* Geneva: Author.

Joint United Nations Program on HIV/AIDS (UNAIDS), United Nations Population Fund (UNFPA), & United Nations Development Fund for Women (UNIFEM). (2004). *Women and HIV/AIDS: Confronting the crisis.* Geneva: Author.

Joint United Nations Program on HIV/AIDS & World Health Organization (UNAIDS & WHO). (2004). *Treats 3 million by 2005: Epidemiological fact sheets on HIV/AIDS and sexually transmitted infections*. China. Geneva: Author.

Kaufman, J., & Jing, J. (2002). China and AIDS-The time to act is now. *Science, 296*, 2339–2340.

Lau, J., & Siah, P. (2001). Behavioral surveillance of sexually related risk behaviours of the Chinese male general population in Hong Kong: A benchmark study. *AIDS Care, 13*, 221–232.

Lau, J., Siah, T., & Tsui, H. (2002). A study of the STD/AIDS related attitudes and behaviours of men who have sex with men in Hong Kong. *Archives of Sexual Behavior, 31*, 367–373.

Ma, S., Duckers, N., van de Hoek, A., Yuliang, F., Zhiheng, C., Jiangting, F., et al. (2002). Decreasing STD incidence and increasing condom use among Chinese sex workers following a short term intervention: A prospective cohort study. *Sexually Transmitted Infections, 78*, 110–114.

Martin, S., & Curtis, S. (2004). Gender-based violence and HIV/AIDS: Recognizing links and acting on evidence. *The Lancet, 363*, 1410–1411.

Pan, S. (2001). *AIDS in China: How much possibility is there in sexual transimitting?* Paper presented at the 1st China Conference on AIDS/STDs, Bejing, China.

Stein, Z. (1990). HIV prevention: The need for methods women can use. *American Journal of Public Health, 80*, 460–462.

Tang, C. (1999). Marital power and aggression in a community sample of Hong Kong Chinese families. *Journal of Interpersonal Violence, 14*, 586–602.

Tang, C. (2006, in press). Gender-based violence in Hong Kong. In F. M. Cheung & E. Holroyd (Eds.), *Mainstreaming gender in Hong Kong society*. Hong Kong: The Chinese University Press.

Tang, C., Wong, C., & Lee, A. (2001). Gender-related psychosocial and cultural factors associated with condom use among Chinese married women. *AIDS Education and Prevention, 14*, 329–342.

Tang, C., Wong, D., & Cheung, F. (2002). Social construction of women as legitimate victims of violence in Chinese societies. *Violence Against Women, 8*, 968–996.

Tucker, J., Henderson, G., Wang, T., Huang, Y., Parish, W., Pan, S., et al. (2005). Surplus men, sex work, and the spread of HIV in China. *AIDS, 19*, 539–547.

Vandeermoortele, J., & Delamonica, E. (2000). Education "vaccine" against HIV/AIDS. *Current Issues in Education, 3*, 1.

Wang, Y. (2000). A strategy of clinical tolerance for the prevention of HIV and AIDS in China. *Journal of Medicine & Philosophy, 25*, 48–61.

Wingood, G., & DiClemente, R. (1996). HIV sexual risk reduction intervention for women: A review. *American Journal of Preventive Medicine, 12*, 209–217.

World Health Organization. (2002). *World report on violence and health*. Geneva: Author.

World Health Organization. (2004). *Women and girls need access to AIDS treatment and protection from violence*. Geneva: Author.

Zhang, K., Li, D., Li, H., & Beck, E. (1999). Changing sexual attitudes and behaviour in China: Implications for the spread of HIV and other sexually transmitted diseases. *AIDS Care, 11*, 581–589.

Knowledge, Attitudes, and Behaviors Related to HIV and AIDS among Female College Students in Taiwan

Wei-Chen Tung
Jie Hu
Cindy Davis
Wei-Kang Tung
Yin-Mei Lin

INTRODUCTION

Despite decades of HIV/AIDS education and prevention programs, almost 5 million people became infected with HIV in 2003, the greatest number in any one year since the beginning of the epidemic (UNAIDS, 2004). Globally, the number of people living with HIV continues to grow with an estimated 38 million people living with HIV in 2003 (UNAIDS). All regions of the world have been touched by this epidemic. The epidemic in Asia is expanding rapidly, with an estimated 7.4 million living with HIV in the region (UNAIDS). Given that Asia is home to 60% of the world's population, the fast-growing Asian epidemic has significant global implications. Several countries in this region are characterized with low per capita incomes, dramatic inequalities in income distribution, and poor health care infrastructures, making it difficult or impossible to deal with the AIDS epidemic (Twu, Huang, Lai, Ming, & Su, 2004).

Taiwan, a democratic island country off the southeast coast of the People's Republic of China, has a population of approximately 23 million people (Lin, Simoni, & Zemon, 2005). In 1986, AIDS was first reported in Taiwan from a male patient who had sex with men (MSM) (Lin et al.). As of early 2006, there were 11,481 cases of HIV infection and 2,581 cases of AIDS reported to the Centers for Disease Control in Taiwan (CDC Taiwan, 2006). Though relatively low compared to other Asian countries, the incidence of HIV infection in Taiwan has increased approximately 15% every year since 1997 (Twu et al., 2004), making this area one of the highest growing rates in Asia (Lin et al.). Demographic data on the HIV-positive population shows that 91% of this population is male, with approximately 30% being homosexual (CDC Taiwan). These data suggest that women in Taiwan are at risk of becoming infected with HIV over the next few years through their male sexual partners.

Early in the epidemic, HIV infection and AIDS were rarely diagnosed in women. Today, the HIV/AIDS epidemic represents a growing and persistent health threat to women, especially young women. As of December 2003, women accounted for nearly 50% of all people living with HIV worldwide (UNAIDS, 2004). Young women are at risk for sexually transmitted HIV for several reasons, including biologic vulnerability, lack of recognition of their partners' risk factors, having sex with older men who are more likely to be infected with HIV, gender norms and the inability to negotiate safer sex practices within the relationship (Centers for Disease Control and Prevention [CDC], 2005). Some women may be unaware of their male partners' risk for HIV infection and may not insist on condom use owing to inequality in the relationship and/or out of fear that their partners will physically abuse them or leave them (Foreman, 2003; Gupta & Weiss, 1993; Suarez-Al-Adam, Raffealli, & O'Leary, 2000). In Taiwanese tradition, women are expected to be submissive to their father at home, their husband after marriage, and their son after the death of the husband (Yeh, 2002). Additionally, while female virginity prior to marriage and fidelity subsequent to marriage are highly valued, men visit a prostitute, which is tolerated within Taiwanese society. Wang and Lin (1996) found that 58% of male partners in Taiwan reported having visited prostitutes; however, fewer than 20% reported ever having used a condom during sexual intercourse with prostitutes. Under the influence of culture on gender roles and males engaging in high-risk sexual behavior, Taiwanese women are even more vulnerable to HIV infection.

Young people between 15 and 24 years of age account for nearly half of all new HIV infections worldwide (UNAIDS, 2004). Young people under the age of 30 make up more than 40% of the HIV-positive population currently reported in Taiwan (CDC Taiwan, 2006). The importance of focusing on young people has been recognized at a global level by the 2001 UN General Assembly Special Session on HIV/AIDS, which endorsed a number of goals for young people, including:

By 2005, ensure that at least 90%, and by 2010 at least 95% of young men and women have access to the information, education, including peer education and youth-specific education, and services necessary to develop the life skills required to reduce their vulnerability to HIV infection; in full partnership with youth, parents, families, educators and health care providers." (WHO, 2000)

College students as a population are particularly vulnerable to HIV infection. Centers for Disease Control and Prevention in a recent report states that the "epicenter of the [HIV/AIDS] epidemic is college students" (CDC, 2004). Incidents of risky sexual behaviors are prevalent among college students, much of which occurs under the influence of drugs and alcohol (CDC, 2004; UNAIDS, 2004). In a sample of Taiwanese college students, Chen (2003) reported that 63% of the respondents had sexual intercourse, with the majority having their first sexual encounter during their college years (Lin et al., 2005). Though Taiwanese are some of the least sexually active people in the world, according to the Global Sex Survey conducted annually by Durex (2005), the prevalence of unprotected sex is greater in Taiwan than in most other Asian countries, with 38% of Taiwanese reportedly having had unprotected sex without knowledge of their partner's sexual history, and the average age of first intercourse was reported at 18.5 years (Lin et al.).

Research on HIV/AIDS knowledge among college students has consistently shown that knowledge alone does not predict safe sex practices (Anastasi, Sawyer, & Pinciaro, 1999; Gupta & Weiss, 1993; Lewis, Malow, & Ireland, 1997; Opt & Loffredo, 2004). According to the Health Belief Model (HBM), the likelihood of engaging in at-risk health behaviors is influenced by attitudes and beliefs that motivate behavior; however, all behaviors are mediated by individual, social, and environmental factors. The HBM hypothesizes that knowledge factors (e.g., perceived susceptibility and perceived severity of a disease) are important to preventing at-risk health behaviors and that these factors are influenced by perceived benefits and barriers to preventative activities. According to the HBM, the likelihood of taking preventative action is determined by one's perceived risk and the sum of pros and cons he or she perceives in taking action; however, many factors may contribute to these assessments.

Given the complexity surrounding one's decision to act responsibility to prevent the transmission of HIV among college students, the purposes of the study were (1) to assess the knowledge and attitudes, source of HIV and AIDS information, and behaviors related to HIV and AIDS among female college students in Taiwan and (2) to explore the factors associated with knowledge and attitudes of HIV and AIDS among female college students in Taiwan.

METHODS

Design and Sample

A descriptive cross-sectional study design was used. A self-administered questionnaire was used to obtain data from female college students. The subjects were recruited from a 4-year university in the southern Taiwan area. Eligible subjects were included if they were (1) aged 18 years or older, (2) able to read Chinese, and (3) female undergraduate students in non-health-related majors.

Data Collection Procedures

Following university ethical approval, a complete list of potential participants' names and addresses was provided for the investigators by the university. Surveys with a self-addressed and stamped return envelope were mailed to 894 female students. A cover letter accompanying the questionnaire explained the purpose of the survey and asked for voluntary participation. Participants were also informed of confidentiality and anonymity. A reminder postcard was sent to students within 3 weeks to increase response rate. The completed questionnaires were returned in a sealed envelope directly to the investigatora and were taken as consent to participate.

Instrument

Demographic Questionnaire. The questionnaire included age, year in school, marital status, income, student status, employment status, health perception, religion, religious level, smoking level, drug use, alcohol use, source of HIV/AIDS information, age at first sexual intercourse, sexually active in the last year, and number of sexual partners during lifetime.

The International AIDS Questionnaire—Chinese Version. The International AIDS Questionnaire—Chinese Version (IAQ-C) (Davis, Tang, Noel, & Chan, 1999) was used to measure HIV/AIDS knowledge and attitudes among female college students in Taiwan. The 18-item IAQ-C assesses four dimensions of HIV and AIDS: transmission myths, facts, attitudes, and personal risk. Each item was scored on a 5-point Likert scale (1 = Strongly Agree, 2 = Agree, 3 = Don't Know, 4 = Disagree, 5 = Strongly Disagree). A total score of the IAQ-C ranges from 18 to 90, and subscales scores range from 7 to 35 for transmission myths, 5 to 25 for attitudes, and 3 to 15 for personal risk and facts. Higher scores indicate positive and accurate views on HIV and AIDS in this study. The IAQ-C total scale had a Cronbach's coefficient alpha of .76 (Davis et al., 1999). The test-retest reliability was accomplished with a sample of 21 Chinese university students at a 2-week interval and was found to be .74. In the present study, the Cronbach's alpha coefficient was .83 for the total 18 items, .90 for the transmission myths subscale, .71 for the attitudes subscale, .55 for the personal risk subscale, and .59 for the facts subscale.

Data Analysis

The data were analyzed using SPSS (Statistical Package for the Social Science) version 12.0 for Windows. The mean, standard deviation, percentage, and frequency distribution were performed to descriptively analyze the demographic variables, the knowledge and attitudes, source of HIV and AIDS information, and behaviors related to HIV and AIDS. Independent t-test and one-way analysis of variance (ANOVA) were used to examine the differences in the total IAQ-C scores among different demographic subgroups (i.e., marital status, student status, employment status, religion, sexually active in the last year, and number of lifetime sexual partners). A post hoc Tukey's test was applied to determine which specific pairs of means differed significantly from one another in the total IAQ-C scores. Pearson's correlation and Spearman's rho were used to evaluate the relationships between the total IAQ-C scores and students' age, year in college, income, health perception, religious level, smoking level, drug use, alcohol use, and age at first sexual intercourse. Reliability analyses were used to measure the internal consistency of the instruments. For all analyses in this research, a level of $p < .05$ was employed to determine statistical significance.

RESULTS

A total of 99 female college students completed the questionnaire and returned it to the investigators, yielding a response rate of 11 %. Table 1 shows the demographic characteristics of the 99 respondents. The mean age of participants was 25.82 (SD = 6.47) years ranging from 18 to 54 years old. Of the 99 participants, most were sophomores (36.4%), were single (62.6%), were working full-time (55.6%), were part-time students (71.7%), and had a religious affiliation (71.7%).

Participants' mean age of having the first sexual experience was at the age of 19.62 (SD = 2.56) ranging from 15 to 28 years. Abut 68.7% of the participants were sexually active in the last year. The average number of sexual partners during lifetime was two ranging from one to four with 46.7% having only one sexual partner and 53.3% having more than two sexual partners.

Knowledge and Attitudes about HIV and AIDS

Sources of HIV/AIDS Information

Eight primary sources of HIV/AIDS information were reported by respondents. Television was the most popular source (73.7%) followed by newspaper (59.6%), health professionals (59.6%), radio (59.6%), Internet (55.6%), school teacher (45.5%), friends (28.3%), and family (18.2%).

IAQ-C Results

Table 2 and Table 3 show the knowledge and attitudes of HIV and AIDS among Taiwanese college female students. The average of all 18 items from the IAQ-C was calculated to indicate general knowledge and attitudes of HIV and AIDS. The mean score of general knowledge and attitudes of HIV and AIDS for all participants was 3.70 (SD = .68). The mean scores of each of four subscales were 4.07 (SD = 1.07) for transmission myths, 3.60 (SD = 1.09) for facts, 3.72 (SD = 1.03) for personal risk, and 3.89 (SD = .74) for attitudes.

Transmission Myths

Findings on HIV/AIDS transmission myths indicated that more than 25% of the participants agreed that mosquitoes can transmit HIV,

TABLE 1. Demographic Characteristics of
Survey Respondents ($N = 99$)

	Number	Percentage
Year in college		
Freshman	23	23.2
Sophomore	36	36.4
Junior	11	11.1
Senior	29	29.3
Marital status		
Single	62	62.6
Married	34	34.3
Divorced	3	3.0
Monthly income[a]		
< NT10000	4	4.4
NT10,001–20,000	3	3.0
NT20,001–30,000	8	8.1
NT30,001–40,000	6	6.1
> NT40,000	16	16.2
Prefer not to say	62	62.6
Student status		
Full time	28	28.3
Part time	71	71.7
Employment status		
Full time job	55	55.6
Part time job	32	32.3
No job	12	12.1
Health perception		
Poor	3	3.0
Fair	50	50.5
Good	25	25.3
Very good	14	14.1
Excellent	7	7.1
Religion		
Buddhist	26	26.3
Christian	20	20.2
Hindi	21	21.2
Shinto	3	3.0
Muslim	1	1.0
None	28	28.3

(continued)

TABLE 1. (*Continued*)

	Number	Percentage
Religious level		
Very religious	28	28.3
Some religious	32	32.3
Little religious	25	25.3
Not at all	14	14.1
Smoking level		
Everyday	8	8.1
Sometimes	26	26.3
Not at all	65	65.7
Drug use		
Occasionally	8	8.1
Not at all	91	91.9
Alcohol use		
Sometimes	58	58.6
Not at all	41	41.4

Note. [a]U.S. $1.00 = NT $32.00.

approximately 23% agreed that swimming pools can spread HIV, 21% agreed that sharing cigarettes can contact HIV/AIDS, 17% agreed that HIV/AIDS can be spread through coughing and sneezing and through the air, 14% agreed that HIV can be contacted through toilet seats, and 12% agreed that hugging an infected person can spread HIV/AIDS.

Facts. Participants' views of factual information on HIV/AIDS revealed that more than 29% of the participants were unaware that condoms would decrease the risk of HIV transmission, 13% were unaware that HIV can be transmitted from mother to baby, and 56.3% were unaware that HIV can be spread through infected sperm.

Personal Risk. Findings on personal risk demonstrated that 31% of the participants agreed that AIDS affected only intravenous drug users, 14% agreed that Asians are less susceptible of contacting to AIDS than Westerners, and 18% believed that vaccination can protect themselves against AIDS.

Attitudes. Participants' attitudes toward AIDS indicated that 24% were unwilling to do volunteer work with AIDS patients. About 23% participants agreed that people with HIV should stay home or in a hospital. Less than 10% of the participants thought that people with HIV should be kept out of school or they would end a friendship if

TABLE 2. HIV and AIDS Knowledge and Attitudes Among Female College Students in Taiwan (*N* = 99)

Item on IAQ-C	Mean[a]	SD
Transmission myths	4.07	1.07
HIV can be spread through coughing and sneezing	4.17	1.43
AIDS can be contacted through sharing cigarettes	3.95	1.50
HIV/AIDS can be spread through hugging an infected person	4.41	1.78
HIV can be transmitted through the air	4.25	1.31
HIV can be spread through swimming pools	3.90	1.40
HIV can be contracted through toilet seats	4.16	1.25
Mosquitoes can transmit HIV	3.67	1.50
Facts	3.60	1.09
Condoms will decrease the risk of HIV*	3.61	1.56
HIV can be transmitted from mother to baby*	4.12	1.32
HIV is spread through infected sperm*	3.08	1.52
Personal risk	3.72	1.03
Asians are less susceptible of contacting AIDS than are Westerners	4.01	1.17
AIDS only affects intravenous (IV) drug users, prostitutes and homosexuals	3.23	1.72
You can protect yourself against AIDS by being vaccinated for it	3.94	1.39
Attitudes	3.89	0.74
People with HIV should be kept out of school	4.27	1.13
Would end my friendship if my friend had AIDS	4.07	1.08
I am willing to do volunteer work with AIDS patients*	3.08	1.06
If a family member contracts HIV he/she should move out	4.31	0.99
People with HIV should stay home or in a hospital	3.75	1.26

Note: [a]Based on 5-point Likert scale format, 1 = Strongly Agree, 2 = Agree, 3 = Don't Know, 4 = Disagree, 5 = Strongly Disagree. Higher scores indicate more positive and accurate views on HIV. *Item scores were revised.

their friend had AIDS or family member who contacted HIV should move out of the home.

Factors Associated with Knowledge and Attitudes of HIV and AIDS

The results from one-way ANOVA and Tukey's post hoc test show that participants working full-time (*M* = 70.31, SD = 9.28) had a

TABLE 3. Total Mean Score of Subscale and IAQ-C
($N = 99$)

	Mean	SD	Range
Transmission myths	28.35	7.58	7–35
Facts	10.80	3.26	3–15
Personal risk	11.06	3.19	3–15
Attitudes	19.16	3.95	5–25
IAQ-C	69.38	11.91	18–90

significantly higher total IAQ-C score than participants working part-time ($M = 61.38$, SD $= 14.49$), F (2, 84) $= 5.43$, $p = .01$.

Independent t-test results show that participants who were sexually active in the last year ($M = 67.26$, SD $= 11.96$) had a significantly higher total IAQ-C score than participants were not sexually active in the last year ($M = 54.50$, SD $= 12.53$), $t = 2.49$, $p = .02$. The IAQ-C dimension of attitudes toward HIV and AIDS revealed a significant difference between participants with different number of sexual partners during lifetime. Those with more than one partner ($M = 19.83$, SD $= 3.63$) had a significantly higher attitudes score than those who had only one partner ($M = 17.83$, SD $= 4.34$), $t = 2.20$, $p = .03$. There were no significant differences in the total IAQ-C scores between marital status subgroups, student status subgroups, religion subgroups, and number of sexual partners during lifetime.

The results of the Spearman's rho suggest that the total IAQ-C scores were significantly and positively related to students' year in college ($r_s(99) = .42$, $p < .01$), indicating that participants who had more years in college were more likely to have positive and accurate views on HIV and AIDS. The total IAQ-C scores were significantly and negatively related to students' smoking level ($r_s(99) = -.31$, $p < .01$), indicating that participants who were smoking less were more likely to have positive and accurate views on HIV and AIDS. There was no significant correlation between the total IAQ-C scores and participants' age income, health perception, religious level, drug use, alcohol use, and age at first sexual intercourse.

DISCUSSION

The aim of the current study were (1) to assess the knowledge and attitudes, source of HIV and AIDS information, and behaviors related to HIV and AIDS among female college students in Taiwan and (2) to explore the factors associated with knowledge and attitudes of HIV and AIDS among female college students in Taiwan. Prior to discussing the results, it is important to consider several limitations of the study. The current study relied on a non-probability sample of Taiwanese college females, which limits the generalizability of the results, especially given the low response rate. Our study attempted to minimize, but could not rule out, the shortcomings of the self-reported method, which may be subject to self-selection, social desirability, and recall bias. Despite these limitations, the results of the study provide important information on HIV and AIDS knowledge and attitudes among college women in Taiwan, which has significant implications for AIDS prevention in this country.

Despite this sample's being a highly educated group of college women in Taiwan, their knowledge of HIV and AIDS information was surprisingly poor. For example, a significant number of the respondents thought that HIV could be transmitted by mosquitoes (25%), swimming pools (23%), sharing cigarettes (21%), coughing or sneezing in the air (17%), toilet seats (14%), and hugging an infected person (12%). Furthermore, more than half the sample was unaware that HIV is spread via infected sperm, and nearly 30% were unaware that condoms would decrease the risk of HIV transmission. Other HIV and AIDS myths held by a significant number of respondents included that AIDS affected only IV drug users (31%) and that a vaccine could prevent AIDS (18%).

The most popular source of HIV and AIDS information was television followed by newspapers, health professionals, radio, internet, and school teachers. Accurate HIV and AIDS information is the first step in preventing the spread of this epidemic. Further analysis of Taiwanese society's stance towards HIV/AIDS, including media representations and government policies would be instructive. Of particular significance would be the provision of accurate HIV and AIDS education in public schools at the secondary and university level, given that fewer than half of the respondents reported teachers as a source of HIV and AIDS information. Earlier studies from Taiwan found that though the textbook includes the reproductive system and sex information, some teachers in secondary schools avoid giving instructions and ask students to read the text for themselves because of teacher's discomfort with the subject of sex (Tsai & Wong, 2003; Yeh, 2002). In recognition of the fact that sex education is not sufficient in schools, Department of Health (DOH) in Taiwan (2006) has launched several campaigns to prevent and control AIDS/HIV by stressing the importance of safe sex. For instance, the DOH has established 33 teen health centers throughout the island, where medical advice, consultation and referral services are provided for teens seeking help or interested in finding out more about safe sex. The DOH also has set up a sex education Web site at http://www.young.gov.tw. This Web site has reached page views of about 500,000 per year—an indication that more and more youths are visiting the site to get information on safe sex or to seek online help. Nevertheless, the inadequacy of formal instructions on sex education has forced youth to depend on informal channels (e.g., Internet and newspaper) and might lead to significant obstacles to a full understanding of safe sex practice. Research has shown that people need a solid factual understanding of HIV and its transmission, access to relevant services and supplies, and the confidence and social power to initiate and sustain behavioral change in order to prevent the spread of HIV and AIDS (Gupta & Weiss, 1993). Ideally, the fight against AIDS should involve the family, education system, mass media, and society at large; however, the lack of necessary knowledge, values and skills often results in ineffective and inconsistent HIV and AIDS prevention programs.

Similar to previous studies on sexual activities among Taiwanese college students (Chen, 2003), our study revealed that the majority of respondents (68%) were sexually active in the last year. Findings revealed that the sexually active women had more overall HIV and AIDS knowledge and attitudes compared to those who were not sexually active. Though knowledge is an essential first step in the fight against HIV and AIDS, previous research of HIV/AIDS knowledge among college students has consistently shown that knowledge alone does not predict safe sex practices (Anastasi et al., 1999; CDC, 2004; Gupta & Weiss, 1993; Lewis et al., 1997; Opt & Loffredo, 2004).

Our study focused on HIV and AIDS knowledge; however, further intervention-based research needs to be conducted on how to increase safe sex practices among this vulnerable population and increase condom self-efficacy. AIDS and HIV prevention programs have been the primary focus of controlling the spread of this disease since the epidemic was discovered, but effective programs require the understanding of the target groups' characteristics, their particular stage of needs, and predicting factors specific to their behavior change. Future studies should focus on further understanding the social, cultural, and psychological factors that hamper safe sex practices among this population as well as successful intervention strategies to overcome these barriers.

REFERENCES

Anastasi, M., Sawyer, R. G., & Pinciaro, P. J. (1999). A descriptive analysis of students seeking HIV antibody testing at a university health service. *Journal of American College Health, 48,* 13–20.

Centers for Disease Control and Prevention (CDC). (2005). Fact Sheet-HIV/AIDS among youth. Retrieved on July 19, 2005, from http://www.cdc.gov/hiv/pubs/facts/youth.htm.

Centers for Disease Control and Prevention. (2004). HIV/AIDS and college students. A CDC pathfinder 1995. Atlanta: Author.

Centers for Disease Control and Prevention, Taiwan. (2006). HIV Epidemiology in Taiwan, 1984-2006, March 31. Retrieved on April 5, 2006, from http://aids.cdc.gov.tw/iscomdms/webupload/9503Monthly%20Report.pdf

Chen, Y. C. (2003). A study on the relationships between sex knowledge, sex ideas and sexual behavior of college students in Great Taipei area. Taiwan: National Central Library.

Davis, C., Tang, C., Noel, M. B., & Chan, F. (1999). The development and validation of the International AIDS Questionnaire—Chinese Version. *Education and Psychological Measurement, 59*(3), 481–491.

Department of Health of the Executive Yuan of Taiwan. (2006). DOH measures to promote safe sex among youth. Retrieved on May 17, 2006, from http://www.doh.gov.tw/NewVersion/Media/SE931001-1.doc

Durex. (2005). Global sex survey. Retrieved on May 9, 2006, from http://www.durex.com/cm/gss2005results.asp

Foreman, F. E. (2003). African American college women: Constructing a hierarchy of sexual arrangements. *AIDS Care, 15*(4), 493–504.

Gupta, G., & Weiss, E. (1993). Women and AIDS: Developing a new health strategy (Policy Series, No. 1). Washington, DC: International Center for Research on Women.

Lewis, J. E., Malow, R. M., & Ireland, S. J. (1997). HIV/AIDS risk in heterosexual college students. A review of a decade of literature. *Journal of the American College of Health, 45*(4), 147–158.

Lin, P., Simoni, J. M., & Zemon, V. (2005). The Health Belief Model, sexual behaviors, and HIV risk among Taiwanese immigrants. *AIDS Education and Prevention, 17*(5), 469–483.

Opt, S. K., & Loffredo, D. A. (2004). College students and HIV/AIDS: More Insights on knowledge, testing, and sexual practices. *Journal of Psychology, 138*(5), 389–402.

Suarez-Al-Adam, M., Raffealli, M., & O'Leary, A. (2000). Influence of abuse and partner hyper-masculinity on the sexual behavior of Latinas. *AIDS Education and Prevention, 12,* 263–274.

Tsai, Y. F., & Wong, T. K. S. (2003). Strategies for resolving aboriginal adolescent pregnancy in eastern Taiwan. *Journal of Advanced Nursing, 41,* 351–357.

Twu, S. J., Huang, Y. F., Lai, A. C., Ming, N., & Su, I. J. (2004). Update and projection on HIV/AIDS in Taiwan. *AIDS Education and Prevention, 16,* 53–63.

UNAIDS. (2004). 2004 Report on the global AIDS epidemic. Geneva: Joint United Nations Programme on HIV/AIDS.

Wang, P. D., & Lin, R. S. (1996). Risk factors for cervical intraepithelial neoplasia in Taiwan. *Gynecologic Oncology, 62,* 10–18.

World Health Organization. (2000). HIV/AIDS and Adolescents. Retrieved on July 27, 2005, from http://www.who.int/child-adolescent-health/HIV/HIV_adolescents. htm.

Yeh, C. H. (2002). Sexual risk taking among Taiwanese youth. *Public Health Nursing, 19,* 68–55.

Fallout from Communism: The Role of Feminism in Fighting HIV/AIDS among Women in Russia

Michael N. Humble
Brian E. Bride

The human immunodeficiency virus (HIV) and the acquired immune deficiency syndrome (AIDS) are considered by many to now be the chronic illnesses in the United States (Dray-Spira & Lert, 2003). Unfortunately, the virus continues to affect the most marginalized communities, especially women of color, though this would be difficult do discern owing to headlines regarding HIV/AIDS's dropping dramatically over the past 10 years because of recent medical advances, such as the triple-combination therapy (AIDS Weekly & Law, 2004). The virus still has a foothold in the United States, but one must look closely to see any evidence in the media of its continued presence. Gone are the days of front-page news stories shouting for urgency regarding recent deaths from AIDS. The Elizabeth Glasers and Ryan Whites have all been overshadowed by almost 10 years of access to life-prolonging drugs. HIV/AIDS in the United States has gone from a hot topic to one that is barely mentioned.

Capitalism born of democracy has made the United States a country rich in resources, at least as compared to many other nations currently battling the spread of HIV/AIDS. Though it is still debatable whether the United States is doing everything possible to prevent the spread of the virus within its own borders, it is not debatable that most underdeveloped countries lack the resources necessary to contain this epidemic. One need look no further than South Africa to see that without proper prevention methods as well as governmental support of these prevention measures, both monetarily and otherwise, HIV/AIDS has the potential to spread at a rapid rate. Even within our own country in which governmental programs and private insurance allow most access to HIV/AIDS treatments, rates of infections continue to rise in contrast to the decline that many thought would happen once prevention messages were spread (Centers for Disease Control and Prevention [CDC], 2006).

While access to treatment for women with HIV/AIDS is on the rise in the United States, The World Health Organization (WHO) (as cited in Grogan, 2006) reported that every region in the world saw an increase in the number of women being infected with HIV/AIDS. Their joint report with the United Nations Program on HIV/AIDS discussed the vulnerability of women and girls in the HIV/AIDS pandemic. The target goal of those in the United Nations and the WHO is access to treatments, treatments that currently are available only to the richest of countries.

One country in which HIV/AIDS has swelled from a trickle to a downpour is in the former Soviet Republics. The Nation's Health (2004) proclaimed that Estonia, Russia, and Ukraine are fighting the highest rate of new infections in the world. Further, they estimated that an average of 1 of every 100 persons in those countries is currently HIV-positive. Even more daunting is the fact that fewer than 10% of those infected have access to proper care and treatment. How could a country that was sold on the principles of socialism and the common good for so many decades have lost its way when dealing with this public health crisis?

EVOLUTION OF RUSSIA TODAY

The late 1980s and early 1990s saw the fall of the Berlin Wall as well as the dissolution of the Soviet Union. Consumerism began to replace communism in quick-time as lives that were once dictated by the government were now dictated by the Eruo. "By the late 1990s, shopping districts in both large cities and small towns displayed an eclectic, postmodern style, combining flashy 'Euro standard' architecture with faded, crumbling, apartment buildings and generic shop fronts more reminiscent of the Soviet period" (Patico & Caldwell, 2002). The facades on store fronts were not the only things that were changing. The experiment known as communism had failed in this part of the world and been replaced with a newer version of democracy (Kovac, 2002).

Traditionally, women in Russia were placed in governmental positions as well as general employment in order to achieve government quotas. Women associated feminism with "primitive stereotypes" (Tevernise, 2003) and saw no need for a movement to empower themselves. Most felt as though they had a government in which feminism was already a built-in mechanism. With the fall of the communist government also came a fall of the traditional roles of women in the country. "The situation for women compared with Soviet times got worse. Most women's organizations are self-help centers. But these problems need to be resolved" (Tavernese, 2003, p. N4). Ianovskii and Perminova (1996) counters the myth of equality of women in the Soviet Union by examining the duality that women were entrenched in, that of working socialist and then coming home to cleaning the house and taking care of children. Though all appeared equal, the communist Soviet Union was experiencing the same types of societal issues regarding the roles and treatment of women as the Western world.

Much has been written about women during the Stalin era (Chatterjee, 2002; Leder, 2002; Simmons & Perlina, 2002), but there is very little mention of the idea of feminism among this body of literature. It is as if feminism was an idea that could not be conceived of during the socialist movement. Since the fall of communism, many social scientists have examined the plight of women in the new Russia (Temkina & Zdravomyslova, 2003; Ianovskii & Perminova, 1996; Sundstrom, 2002). This new dialogue seems to embrace the theoretical model of feminism when examining roles of women in this new democracy. This literature uses the lens of feminism to try to understand how the roles of women have changed so dramatically over the past 15 years.

Multiple books (Cohen, 2000; Cox, 1998; Reddaway & Glinski, 2001) have chronicled the fall of communism in Russia. Most of these have included a critique on the West's involvement in this new democracy. The theme that is apparent in all of these critical examinations is that the new Russia has failed on many different levels. Not terribly, but none the less, the former Soviet Union has had a tough ride in its transformation from Bolshevism to capitalism. Pope (1991) observed the victims of communism's fall, those involved in government, and prophesized a new Russia that would not discriminate against those who were involved in the socialist movement.

Ruchkin (2000) reported that the youth of the new Russia are disillusioned about the prospects for the future. Ruchkin went on to say that "the strata of the working class and the peasantry, differences are becoming deeper with respect to income and economic and political interests" (p. 57). This author also stated the ever-increasing divorce rates as another reason for disdain. Reports have also shown that health is deteriorating at a drastic and much faster rate than the previous generation. Along with this disparity in health care is the depopulatization the country is experiencing. With two of every five pregnancies ending in abortion, many in government fear they will not have enough people to keep the slow moving economy going (Ruchkin).

Social work's role in this transformation has also not escaped notice. Templeman (2001) discussed the various social issues that have now brought the development of the profession of social work into the new Russia. Though the first formal social work training program was established in Moscow in 1991, efforts to establish services that would help families dealing with poverty, substance use, and public health epidemics have been difficult to conceive. Templeman stated, "The transition from communism to democracy has brought the recognition and acknowledgment of long-standing social problems, an increase in human struggles and the creation of new dilemmas" (p. 97). One of the greatest dilemmas that this part of the world is currently dealing with is the rapid rate of new HIV/AIDS infections.

What do we really know about a country that was shrouded in mystery for so many decades? Leitzel (1997) proclaimed we know very little:

This lack of consensus is fueled by several factors. First, statistical shortcomings make it difficult to actually gauge the current state of affairs. Standard socio-economic indicators provide only a narrow glimpse into the life of any society, but the view is singularly Cycolopean and distorted in transitional socialist countries. There seems to be a larger unrecorded sector in Russia than in most Western market economies., for example, reducing the reliability of output and income indicators. (p. 49)

What then can we hope to find out about the current state of HIV/AIDS in Russia? This is a country that prided itself on keeping its doors closed to all outsiders. Though this seemed to have worked during the early days of the epidemic, one has to wonder whether the public health procedures were in place to properly document the spread of the virus. Further, if the procedures are in place now, who is monitoring it?

HIV/AIDS AND RUSSIA

The Institute of Medicine (IOM) reported (as cited in Bobrova, Sergeev, Grechukhina, & Kapiga, 2005) that though women were only a small group being affected by the early days of the epidemic, they are now the fastest-growing group of new infections. The high rate of infections is due to multiple factors such as sexual subordination, economic subordination, and female vulnerability to HIV/AIDS (IOM, 2005). The best protection thus far appears to be microbicides, gels, and creams that will help protect women during sexual intercourse. This veritable miracle cream could be available as soon as 2010. None too soon, according to studies that explored gender roles of women in Europe and vulnerability toward HIV/AIDS infection (Kelly, Bobo, Avery, & McLachlan, 2004).

With the first documented case of AIDS in 1987, HIV was a late arrival in Russia largely owing to the country's isolation during the Soviet period (Bigg, 2005). Unfortunately, the country has more than made up for the lost time. With estimates of 1.5 million living with HIV/AIDS and fewer than 10% having access to triple combination therapy, the new Russia is experiencing an overload of HIV/AIDS (Radio Free Europe, 2005). Bobrova, Sergeev, Grechukhina, and Kapiga (2005) estimated that not only does Russia have one of the highest rates of new infections, the majority of these new infections are occurring in adolescents and younger adults. Their study of condom use among young people in Moscow demonstrated that consistent condom use was relatively low among sexually experienced youth in that city. They lobbied for not only condom promotion programs but an overall increase of sexual awareness in a country that until 15 years ago had labeled sex a taboo subject.

Aris and Clark (2004) reported that rampant drug abuse, as well as high levels of poverty, were the building blocks for the dramatic spread of HIV/AIDS across the New Russia. Further, they stated that Russia's new infections are spreading faster than any other European nation, becoming one of the country's most ominous public health crises. Grogan (2006) agreed with this sentiment in her report on substance use in Russia in which she stated that "UNICEF attributes much of this increase to high levels of intravenous drug use among young people" (p. 569). Aris and Clark stated that this IV drug–using population has bridged the epidemic from an exclusive core group out into the general population. Gore-Felton et al (2003) explored the issue of gender on HIV/AIDS risk among intravenous drug users in Russia. By examining gender roles, the authors concluded,

> As Russia and the former Soviet republics endure rising rates in HIV/AIDS, syphilis, gonorrhea, and other STDs, understand the risks among populations where the epidemic is hitting the hardest is critical to the development and implication of effective HIV/AIDS prevention programs. Our study indicates that gender is an important factor in predicting sexual risk behavior associated with multiple sexual partners, both as an independent predictor and a moderating factor. (p. 889)

Montagne (citing National Public Radio [NPR], 2006) stated that the United Nations is not having much success in curbing the spread of HIV/AIDS in the former Soviet Union. The government has promised to increase spending, but most of the fight against the spread, much like the United States during the Reagan years, seems to be taking place at the grass roots level. One organization has even begun to hold a yearly beauty contest for HIV-positive contestants. The reason for this pageant is twofold: first to increase public awareness of the virus and second to break down stereotypes about those who are infected.

Much like the virus, stereotypes and fear about HIV/AIDS seem to be rampant across all of New Russia. Stories about discrimination from health care workers and unfriendly neighborhoods are reminiscent of the epidemic here in the United States during the 1980s. "Experts say the severe stigma and discrimination HIV/AIDS suffers face in Russia is particularly damaging in the case of children" (Bigg, 2005, p. 2). The New Russia is experiencing some growing pains in the area of acceptance and knowledge of the HIV/AIDS virus. But not all of the news is so bleak. The Ukraine region (Malyuta, Newell, Ostergren, Thorne, & Zhilka, 2006) had some promising results from a program that offered voluntary testing and therapy to newly pregnant women. This study showed that nearly 97% of women volunteered to be tested for HIV/AIDS, with those who tested positive being started on triple combination therapy.

The problem of HIV/AIDS in the newly westernized world of the former Soviet Union is reminiscent of the public perception of the virus in the United States before Magic Johnson and triple combination therapy. Though all are at risk in that region of the world for infections, it appears as though women, owing to societal norms, are particularly vulnerable to new infection. What was lacking in the Soviet Union prior to the collapse of communism could be the very tool that is needed now to empower women in the fight against HIV/AIDS: feminism.

FEMINISM AND HIV/AIDS

Today's world is driven by those who have the economic power to feed it. All others take a backseat to the producers in society. What is born of the interactions between owners of production and consumers is capitalism. "Capitalism is organized so that the ruling class comes to own the products of the proletariat's (members of the working class) labor, and so capitalism causes workers to feel cut off from their work and to lack a sense of meaning in their work lives" (Saulnier, 1996, p. 54). Though Marx's overarching theory did not account for gender, socialist feminism has filled that gap. Socialist feminism is aimed at describing the plight of women with regard to today's economic world culture.

Though social feminism speaks to the economic plight of women, liberal feminism is more encompassing as it seeks to explore the social injustices, beyond economic, that women face in today's world. Traditionally, liberal feminists align themselves with the belief that equal rights of women in today's society are restricted by the fact that women are oppressed as a group and do not hold the same rights as men (Saulnier, 1996). Further, until women experience political and financial equality with men, their plight will remain largely unchanged (Enslin & Tjattas, 2004).

The idea of social inequalities putting women at greater risk for HIV/AIDS is nothing new (Zierler & Krieger, 1997). But what about the idea of feminism used as a tool in a country that for decades was living under the assumption that feminism was an ideal that meant nothing to them. Could the touchstones that fuel feminism transfer to a country once rooted in communism and now being showered with democracy?

Non-governmental agencies (NGOs) in the new Russia have proliferated, thanks to foreign grant money. Though these agencies seek to combat many of the ills the country is experiencing, they have not been able to tackle the multiple problems faced by women in that country. One would think that the new NGO's could spark a women's movement, but instead,

> Given their money problems and extent of inequalities between men and women in Russia, we might expect a successful women's movement to grow on the basis of serious grievances. Ample scholarly work exists, both Russian and Western, that documents the unequal status and opportunities of women compared with those of men in Russia. (Sundstrom, 2002, p. 208)

Instead, the movement seems to be stalled in lack of leadership as well as political influence. Though these NGO's have helped communication between leaders of the women's movement, they has not provided the springboard as hoped. Though the country is attempting to tackle issues America has been dealing with for decades, such as violence and sexual inequalities, they are having a difficult time finding a feminist voice to lead them (Hemment, 2004).

How would liberal feminists address the problem of women in the new Russia who are experience astronomical rates of new HIV/AIDS infections? How could they have an impact on a world in which women will not ask their boyfriends about previous sexual partners or the track marks on their arms?

> Prevention programs, whether they focus on substance abuse, pregnancy, or STDs seldom acknowledge a conflict between culturally determined gender norms such as politeness or conformity and the assertive behaviors expected by the program. To move from a position of received knowledge to one of constructed knowledge in which they recognize and communicate opinions, thoughts, and needs, girls and women need to actively participate in environments that assist them in developing their own voice and life direction. (Kelly, et al., 2004, p. 129)

Liberal feminism is concerned with economic access, political equality, education, and reproductive rights to name a few (Saulnier, 1996). One of the overarching themes that seem to be wreaking havoc among the liberal feminists is the dilemma regarding special rights. While some acknowledge that special benefits for women are still very much needed, others say it detracts from the strides women have made and, further, leaves the door open for men to claim women are inferior. Much as with the racial and economic inequalities that exist globally, the world has not come to a time when women are treated on the same plane as men. Therefore, special rights are crucial in the fight against HIV/AIDS with regard to women. This right can be the difference between life and death in a country such as the new Russia in which programs are scattered and prevention messages sparse. Liberal feminists in the new Russia must lobby for more prevention money to be spent on young women, not just dollars that preach abstinence but dollars that preach self-esteem and self-worth. If the new Russia were able to increase feminism, would the outlook for women appear so bleak? Would a unified sense of social justice among Eastern Europe's new women being raised in a capitalistic, democratic society somehow give them the skills to avoid HIV/AIDS infection?

FUTURE OUTLOOK

Russia has the potential to become a great democracy. Unfortunately, this has not happened yet. The early days after the fall of communism saw great prosperity for some but even greater turmoil for most. A country that had prided itself on taking care of its own was thrust into a world in which everyone took what they could and left soon after.

Women in the new Russia are faced with multiple obstacles in order to survive. In a country in which poverty and a lack of social service programs inhibit most, women are especially hard hit. The New Russia has three of five babies aborted. Based on this fact alone, it would seem that the new Russia lacks many of the political constraints that the United States faces when combating HIV/AIDS. In the liberal environment of the New Russia, it would seem that HIV/AIDS education and prevention efforts could flourish. This is the time to seize the opportunity to impart sexual education for women across the new Russia.

Public health efforts must be unified in order to assist the grassroots movements that are already distributing education. The world has the opportunity to take part in the re-education of HIV/AIDS cases in this region. Unfortunately, history has not shown that the rest of the world is concerned with rates of HIV/AIDS infections in countries battling the virus. These same countries usually lack the infrastructure to provide treatment that would help enhance quality of life. The new

Russia is not the exception but the rule when it comes to developing nations and how they are coping with HIV/AIDS. The new global world has had many opportunities to help curb the spread of HIV/AIDS in a variety of different locations. The new Russia is one such area that could benefit from long-term goals regarding treatment and prevention of HIV/AIDS/AIDS. Women in this region are particularly vulnerable and could benefit from some of the ideals embedded in liberal feminism. Perhaps if these values could be infused into programs currently assisting women, these same women would be given the gifts of self-esteem and education that would transfer into an avoidance of the HIV/AIDS epidemic.

REFERENCES

AIDS Weekly & Law. (2004, April 12). HIV/AIDS/AIDS awareness: Media coverage of HIV/AIDS/AIDS decreasing, but focus on global epidemic increasing. Retrieved September 3, 2005, from Lexis-Nexis Academic Universe database.

Aris, B., & Clark, T. (2004, December 4). Russia confronts the threat of AIDS. Retrieved www.thelancet.com, vol. 364.

Bigg, C. (2005, November 30). Russia: HIV strikes hard at young women, children. Radio Free Europe/Radio Liberty, pp. 1–3.

Bobrova, N., Sergeev, O., Grechukhina, T., & Kapiga, S. (2005). Social-cognitive predictors of consistent condom use among young people in Moscow. *Perspectives on Sexual and Reproductive Health, 37*(4), 174–178.

Chatterjee, C. (2002). *Celebrating women: Gender, festival culture, and Bolshevik ideology, 1910–1939*. Pittsburgh: University of Pittsburg Press.

Cohen, S. F. (2000). *Failed crusade: America and the tragedy of post-communist Russia*. London: W.W. Norton.

Cox, M. (Ed.). (1998). *Rethinking the Soviet collapse: Sovietology, the death of communism and the new Russia*. London: Pinter.

Dray-Spira, R., & Lert, F. (2003). Social health inequalities during the course of chronic HIV disease in the era of highly active anti-retroviral therapy. *AIDS, 17*, 283–290.

Enslin, P., & Tjiattas, M. (2004). Liberal feminism, cultural diversity and comparative Education. *Comparative Education, 40*(4), 503–516.

Gore-Felton, C., Somlai, A. M., Benotsch, E. G., Kelly, J. A., Ostrovski, D., & Kozlov, A. (2003). The influence of gender on factors associated with HIV/AIDS transmission risk among young Russian injections drug users. *The American Journal of Drug and Alcohol Abuse, 29*(4), 881–894.

Grogran, L. (2006). Alcoholism, tobacco, and drug use in the countries of central and eastern Europe and the former Soviet Union. *Substance Use & Misuse, 41*, 567–571.

Hemment, J. (2004). Global civil society and the local costs of belonging: Defining violence against women in Russia. *Journal of Women in Culture and Society, 29*(3), 815–840.

Ianovskii, R. G., & Perminova, A. I. (1996). Women and society in Russia. *Russian Social Science Review, 37*(5), 3–10.

Jefferson, D. (2006, May 15). How AIDS changed America. *Newsweek, CXLVII*(20), 36–41.

Kelly, J. P., Bobo, T., Avery, S., & McLachlan, K. (2004). Feminist perspectives and practice with young women. *Issues in Comprehensive Pediatric Nursing, 27,* 121–133.

Klein, L.R., & Pomer, M. (Eds.). (2001). *The new Russia: Transition gone awry.* Stanford: Stanford University Press.

Kovac, L. (2002). The failure of communism: A case for evolutionary rationalism and evolutionary humanism. *Dialogue and Universalism, 8*(10), 177–196.

Leder, M. (2002). *My life in Stalinist Russia: An American women looks back.* Bloomington: Indiana University Press.

Leitzel, J. (1997). Lessons of the Russian economic transition. *Problems of Post-Communism, 44*(1), 49–58.

Malyuta, R., Newell, M. L., Ostergren, M., Thorne, C., & Zhilka, N. (2006). Prevention of mother-to-child transmission of HIV infection: Ukraine experience to date. *European Journal of Public Health, 16*(2), 123–127.

Montagne, R. (2006, May 18). Russia increases budget to battle AIDS. NPR "Morning Edition."

Patico, J., & Caldwell, M. L. (2002). Consumers exiting socialism: Ethnographic perspectives on daily life in post-communist Europe. *Ethnos, 67*(3), 285–294.

Pope, V. (1991). The victims of communism's fall. *U. S. News & World Report, 111*(11), 30–32.

Reddaway, P., & Glinski, D. (2001). *The tragedy of Russia's reforms: Market bolshevism against democracy.* Washington DC: United States Institute of Peace Press.

Ruchkin, B.A. (2000). Youth and the emergence of the new Russia. *Russian Social Science Review, 41*(4), 56–73.

Saulnier, C. F. (1996). *Feminist theory and social work: Approaches and applications.* New York: The Haworth Press.

Simmons, C., & Perlina, N. (Eds.). (2002). *Writing the siege of Leningrad: Women's diaries, memoirs, and documentary prose.* Pittsburg: University of Pittsburg Press.

Sundstrom, L. M. (2002). Women's NGOs in Russia: Struggling from the margins. *Demokratizatsiya, 10*(2), 207–229.

Tavernise, S. (2003, March 9). Women redefine their roles in the new Russia. *New York Times,* p. N4.

Temkina, A., & Zdravomyslova, E. (2003). Gender studies in post-Soviet society: western frames and cultural differences. *Studies in Eastern Thought, 55,* 51–61.

Templeman, S. B. (2001). Social work in the new Russia at the start of the millennium. *International Social Work, 47*(1), 95–107.

The Nation's Health (2004, April). HIV/AIDS soaring in former Soviet republics, Eastern Europe. p. 18.

Zierler, S., & Krieger, N. (1997). Reframing women's risk: Social inequalities and HIV/AIDS infection. *Annual Review Public Health, 18,* 401–436.

Culturally Grounded HIV Prevention for Latino Adolescents in Border Areas: Rationale, Theory, and Research

Rodney A. Ellis
Lori K. Holleran-Steiker
Samuel A. MacMaster
Laura Hopson
Debra Nilson

The face of the HIV/AIDS epidemic has changed over the past decade, as has the face of the U.S. population. Although the disease has remained consistently deadly, it has sought new groups to invade, leaving the once-dominant perception that it is a "gay disease" far behind. During this same period, the nation's ethnic composition has changed, driven by the twin forces of immigration and domestic birth rate. The quantity and distribution of persons of various ethnicities has shifted, and HIV/AIDS has increased disproportionately among some of these groups.

As these processes have persisted, the need for culturally effective prevention and intervention strategies has outstripped the knowledge and skill of many service providers. Further, homelessness has increased, and with it have come changes in the patterns of use of a variety of illicit substances. These conditions present even greater challenges to the social work professional. The challenges are compounded among some groups because of historical and political factors that have lead them to distrust social service providers. The result has been limited contact with service providers and a subsequent exclusion for members of many groups from access to a comprehensive array of services. Further, even when resources have been accessed, cultural dissimilarities between providers and service recipients have limited the effectiveness of interventions. The combined effects of isolation from social services and cultural ineffectiveness of services argue convincingly for the development of culturally-grounded interventions. This article provides a summary of the rationale, theory, and empirical results that support the importance of the development of culturally grounded interventions, particularly for use in HIV prevention programs. A specific example, that of Mexican adolescents residing along the U.S.-Mexican border, is used to underscore these points.

RATIONALE: THE INTERACTIVE EFFECTS OF DIVERSITY, RISK, AND AGE

The number of Latinos residing in the United States has risen, and continues to rise. Data from the 2000 U.S Census indicate that 35.5 million Latinos (12% of the total population) live in the United States. Between 1990 and 2000, the number of Latinos grew from 22.4 million to 35.3 million (a 58% increase), a rate five times greater than for any other ethnicity (Guzman, 2001). Additional estimates indicate that by 2050 Latinos will constitute 24.4% of the population. In contrast, whites are expected to experience a proportional decrease (from 81.0% to 72.1%) and African-Americans are expected to experience a moderate increase, from 12.7% to 14.6% (U.S. Census Bureau, 2004). It is important to note that Latinos have disproportionately low incomes (23% are below the poverty line) and low levels of education (Therrien & Ramirez, 2000).

Latinos in the United States have arrived from a variety of sources. Persons of Mexican descent comprise the largest group. The last decade has seen an influx of immigrants from countries such as Nicaragua, Salvador, Colombia, Venezuela, and the Dominican Republic. This trend is reflected in the 97% increase among such groups reported by 2000 U.S Census. About three-fourths of American Latinos live in four states: Florida, California, New York, and Texas (Guzman, 2001), with a substantial number residing along the U.S.-Mexico border.

Although Latinos are viewed collectively for census purposes, substantial differences often exist between and among subgroups. Factors such as diversity of geographical origin, immigration experience, differential experience of oppression, and area of current residence have a powerful influence on individuals and groups (Ellis, Klepper, and Sowers, 2000a). In fact, Silva (1983) identified five life dimensions that interact within individual experiences to produce diversity. These dimensions are (1) inherited endowment, (2) learned values and culture, (3) developmental histories, (4) specified patterns of problems, and (5) personalized styles of coping. Although certain similarities often exist across Latino subgroups, differential experiences among these life dimensions have produced significant diversity as well. This diversity has important implications for intervention with persons of Latino descent (Atkinson, Morten, & Wing Sue, 1998; Ellis, Klepper, and Sowers, 2000b).

HIV/AIDS Risk Among Latinos

HIV infection is disproportionately high among U.S. Latinos. For instance, although in 2001 Latinos constituted 13% of the total population, they represented 19% of the new HIV cases. The primary means through which the disease is contracted varies from that of the dominant group. AIDS surveillance data indicate that Latino males are more likely to be exposed through injection drug use than non-Hispanic white men. Latina women are more likely to be exposed through sexual encounters than non-Hispanic white women (CDC, 2002).

The literature reports a clear correlation between high rates of HIV infection and high-risk behaviors associated with injection drug use. It is unclear, however, whether this is applicable to all Latinos or to specific subgroups such as Mexican Americans. Frank (2000) found an increase in injection drug use among young Latinos. Increased rates of injection drug use would logically contribute to increased rates of HIV infection, given that injection drug use accounts for more than a third of diagnosed AIDS cases among Latinos (Centers for Disease Control [CDC], 2002). Studies including analysis of Latino subgroups, however, suggest that this may be more reflective of Puerto Ricans than Latinos as a group. Injection drug use has historically played a more central role in HIV infection among Puerto Ricans than among other Latino groups (COSSMHO, 1991).

Several factors have been identified as contributory to Latino representation among those infected with HIV (CDC, 2002). These include poverty, low educational achievement, and limited access to health care. The demographics of Latinos in the Southwest suggest that these factors may play a more central role than does the use of injected substances. As of March, 2002, two in five Latinos in this area aged 25 or older had not graduated from high school (Ramirez and de la Cruz, 2003). In addition, 8.1% of Latino adults were unemployed as compared to 5.1% of non-Hispanic whites, and 21.4% of Latinos lived in poverty as compared to 7.8% of non-Hispanic whites. Latinos also had low rates of heath insurance coverage as compared to non-Hispanic whites, African-Americans, and Asians (Bhandari, 2004).

Specific sexual behaviors may also contribute to the disparities in HIV rates. Latinas have been found to be at higher risk for exposure to a sexually transmitted disease (STD) through sexual contact than other women (Finer, Darroch, & Singh, 1999). This may be related to cultural norms around condom use. Studies comparing African-

Americans, whites, and Latinos have found Latinas to be less likely to report consistent use of condoms (Sly, Quadagno, Harrisson, Everstein, & Richman, 1997; O'Donnell, O'Donnell, & Stueve, 2001). The latter study also found a younger age for initial sexual contact and less frequent use of birth control. Additionally, Mexican-Americans have been found to be more likely to associate alcohol with risky sexual behaviors (Neff, Crawford, & MacMaster, 2002).

Substantial evidence demonstrates that important differences exist between Latino youth on the U.S.-Mexican border and other Latinos. The differential culture, context, and experiences of these youth suggest a need for alternative approaches to HIV prevention. Yet both program development and research into effective prevention for this group are characterized by their paucity.

The 1,200-mile Texas-Mexico border is one of the poorest and fastest-growing regions of the country. It has more than 2 million residents, 85% Hispanic. Counties on the border have a lower percentage of residents with a high-school diploma and higher poverty rates than the rest of Texas. Residents of these communities also possess unique assets, however. A high percentage of families include two parents, and families often place a high priority on their children's education (U.S. Census Bureau, 2002). Hispanic youth living on the border also demonstrate greater adherence to cultural values and beliefs than those living in other parts of the state. These assets can be used to promote resiliency and to reduce risk for problems such as school failure and drug use (McQueen, Getz, & Bray, 2003).

Summarizing the Rationale for Culturally Grounded Programming

The rationale for culturally grounded programming includes evidence from census data, HIV-infection data, cross-cultural research, and diversity research. In summary, the growing proportion of persons of Latino descent in the United States and the rate of HIV infection among them suggests the importance of effective prevention programs for that group. The demographic and cultural characteristics that have lead to the development of culturally-relevant treatment for specific groups also offer evidence of its importance for prevention. Further, the differential experiences of individuals within groups that are often considered collectively (such as Latinos) may require more individualized consideration when prevention programs are developed.

Theory, Practice, and Outcome: Evidence from Human Behavior and Program Evaluation

The argument for the importance of culturally grounded intervention is informed by, but not restricted to, current theory and knowledge of the behavior of adolescents generally, as well as that of specific ethnic groups. Evidence can also be found in the literature presenting the results of outcome research into past and current prevention programs.

Adolescent HIV Risk. Recent declines in the overall incidence of HIV/AIDS in the general population are not evident among juveniles (CDC, 2002). The number of cases has increased among those between 13 and 24 years old. The number of heterosexual adolescents with HIV/AIDS has also increased (CDC, 2003c). The prevalence of risk behaviors among American teens raises concern about continued vulnerability to the disease. In the United States, youth are more likely to have intercourse by age 16 than those in other Western industrialized countries. They also report having multiple sexual partners, putting them at greater risk (Alan Guttmacher Institute, 2002). Almost half of American high-school students report that they have had sex (more than 7% before the age of 13), and more than a third say they are currently sexually active. Among sexually active students, more than 14% report having had at least four sexual partners, and only 63% percent said they used condoms when they last had intercourse. Because substance use increases the likelihood of risky behavior, it is disturbing that more than 25% used drugs or alcohol before their last sexual intercourse (CDC, 2003c).

Although those infected with HIV during adolescence are often undiagnosed until adulthood, the high rates of other STDs among adolescents raises concern. Women between 15 and 19 years of age represent the largest proportion of women diagnosed with gonorrhea at a rate of about 635 cases per every 100,000. The infection rate for gonorrhea among male adolescents is about 466 per every 100,000 males between ages 15 and 19. The Adolescent Women Reproductive Health Monitoring Project estimates that more than 11% of adolescent women are infected with Chlamydia (CDC, 2003a). The high rate of prevalence of these STDs may suggest the rate of HIV infection is also very high.

Adolescent Substance Use. Substance abuse and HIV risk are closely related because risky sexual behavior is often correlated with drug use. It has become a de facto norm for adolescents to experiment with substances (Kaplow, Curran, & Dodge, 2002). The majority of adolescents in the United States will have used mood-altering substances sometime during their teen years. The Monitoring the Future survey reported that 78.4% of high-school seniors had tried alcohol and 53% had tried an illicit drug (Johnston, O'Malley, & Bachman, 2003a). Almost a third (29%) had tried some drug other than marijuana. These figures have been reasonably consistent since the survey's inception in 1975 (Johnston, O'Malley, & Bachman, 2003b). The Youth Risk Behavior Survey provides similar results, finding that 78% of high-school youths had experimented with alcohol and that (47%) had a drink within the prior month (CDC, 2003b).

Although the rate of substance use among adolescents can be disturbing, it is important to understand that it does not have negative consequences for many. Many limit their experience to a few incidents of experimentation (Kaplow, Curran, & Dodge, 2002). Longitudinal studies suggest that many who use more often during their youth "mature out" of substance use as they assume adult roles and responsibilities (Bachman, Wadsworth, O'Malley, Johnston, & Schulenberg, 1997; Labouvie, 1996). Further, Shedler and Block (1990) found that adolescents who experimented with drugs (did not abstain or adopt abusive patterns) experienced higher levels of good psychological health and were better adjusted than their peers. Clearly, the use of illicit substances is an accepted part of many subcultures of adolescents. This is not to say that experimentation or moderate use is desirable or that it should be supported by social work professionals. Yet it is critical to prevention planning to understand that many youth are a part of a subculture in which their peers regard substance abuse as acceptable. Some are also a part of families in which parents and siblings regard it as acceptable. It is important to remember, however, that most adolescents emerge from their period of experimentation without substantial negative consequences.

Still, despite positive outcomes for some, substance abuse constitutes a substantial risk for a myriad of other difficulties for many adolescents. A convincing number of studies have clearly documented both causal and correlational relationships with a multitude of other problem behaviors, including delinquent and subsequent criminal behavior, school dropout or failure, and severe psychological and emotional issues. Adolescent substance abuse has been documented as a gateway to social and economic underachievement as an adult and as an initiatory process into behavioral patterns that, in many cases, will persist for a lifetime (Jessor & Jessor, 1977; Kandel, 1982; Lerner & Vicary, 1984; Robins, 1980; Shedler & Block, 1990). Most relevant to this article, the use of illicit substances also increases the probability that the user may become infected with the HIV virus. Little, unfortunately, is currently known about the specific manner in which substance use impacts adolescents of Mexican descent residing in border areas.

Substance Use and HIV Risk within the Context of Adolescent Development. An additional factor that must be considered to understand adolescent substance abuse is its relationship to developmental processes. One of the more important of these is the development of the self concept. Adolescent development involves biology, culture, and psychology. Archambault (1992) observes that adolescents are thrust into this period of change by culture and biology. Often, regardless of how well they have been prepared, their sense of self and worth is unsure at best (Lawson & Lawson, 1992: 11). Logically, then, it is reasonable to assume that differences in culture and inherited traits, influenced by environment and the other life dimensions identified by Silva (1983) would produce important difference in both processes and outcomes among and between different groups. For example, a youth whose parents immigrated to this country as Kurdish refugees from Iraq is likely to differ in many important ways from Latino youths whose families have migrated across the U.S.-Mexican border within the past few generations. Similarly, third-generation Cuban youths who are descended from members of the first wave of Cuban youths into Florida are likely to have key characteristics that diverge from those of these border youth.

One of the developmental tasks of adolescence is the progression toward separation and individuation through a shift from primary closeness with parents. This shift is accompanied by increasing intimacy with peers (Savin-Williams & Berndt, 1990). This alteration in importance and intensity of peer relations affects the level of influence peers have on each other regarding substance use. Researchers have identified peer influence as one of the strongest risk factors for substance abuse among majority and minority youth (Beauvais, 1992, 1998).

Adolescents create themselves by trying on new selves and by associating with groups of peers that reflect who they are and want to be. Eccles and Barber (1999) have investigated the types of activities in which youth engage in order to assume the persona of the person they want to be. This persona, or self-schema, influences the meaning of engaging in risky behaviors. The Eccles and Barber study found that a group of high-school students active in student activities and organized school athletics tended to have high alcohol use, yet they were doing well in school and had a high likelihood of going to college. In comparison, a second group that consumed similar amounts of alcohol was engaged in other high-risk behaviors and were doing poorly in school. A third group reported high levels of anxiety beginning around the sixth grade. This group became increasingly anxious as they proceeded through school and increased their drinking, presumably to calm the anxiety. The meaning of alcohol use and the relevant consequences are different for each of these groups. Eccles and Barber (1999) pointed out that telling the first group of young people that alcohol use would have dire consequences for them might be ineffective because their experiences contradict this message. For them, encouraging designated drivers and other tactics to avoid negative consequences might be more effective than abstinence. Clearly, the self-identities and substance use patterns of the other two groups place many of their members at greater risk for poor short and long-term outcomes.

Researchers have identified three reasons adolescents use substances as a part of their identity formation. One reason is that the substances provide a sense that they will understand themselves and their environment better. A second possibility is that they hope to increase their breadth of experience and level of activity. Third, for some it produces a "high" or sense of social ease (Segal, Cromer, Hobfoll, & Wasserman, 1982). Understanding a juvenile's motivation for substance use can be important to effective prevention. Yet the degree to which these or other motivations exist for specific population subgroups such as border-residing Mexican-Americans is currently unknown.

Traditional Substance Abuse Prevention Models

Empirical research into the outcomes of various prevention programs provides both evidence for the importance of culturally grounded intervention and suggestions as to what the components of such intervention might be. The close relationship between substance abuse and HIV infection suggests that a review of the outcome literature for both could be instructive.

Historically, substance abuse prevention has most commonly consisted of information education. This assumes once adolescents are aware of the health hazards of substances they will develop anti-drug attitudes and subsequently choose not to use. Research examining the effectiveness of "information only" prevention programs (Botvin, Baker, & Dusenbury, 1995; Bukoski, 1985; Tobler, 1986, 1989) has found that they fail to produce a reduction in use. In fact, some programs were associated with an increased use (Falck & Craig, 1988). For example, Drug Abuse Resistance Education (DARE), the most widespread drug prevention program in the United States ("Project DARE," 1990), has sometimes not only failed to reduce use but has preceded an increase in substance use (Clayton, 1991; Harmon, 1993).

Social theorists, such as Bandura (1977), Jessor and Jessor (1975, 1977), and McGuire (1974), offer some insight into such failures. Their models consider the complex interplay of individual, social, and environmental factors on adolescent behavior. The ecological model, for instance, stresses the concept of multiple levels of influence on child development and the complex interaction of juvenile and environment (Lorion, 1987; Tolan, Guerra, & Kendall, 1995). Certainly, the risks associated with substance abuse might serve as a deterrent to some juveniles. Yet many are confronted with multiple messages from a variety of social and environmental sources. Parents or friends may use drugs and inform youths that the warnings are overblown and may provide positive reinforcement by demonstrating that the use of illicit substances provides pleasure. Teens who may find messages from their peers that they must use drugs in order to fit in may find those messages more compelling than a prevention program's warning. For some groups, the use of drugs may serve as a statement of manhood or machismo. The importance of a demonstration of one's virility may be a very powerful motivator within some ethnic groups.

Other program components have proven useful in prevention programming. The Substance Abuse and Mental Health Services Administration (SAMHSA) has identified the core components of a number of empirically tested programs. These elements include (SAMHSA, 2002):

(1) Program content addressing life skills or knowledge and skills related to substances (noting that substance-related content alone is inadequate)
(2) Opportunities to practice/use new knowledge
(3) Community building beyond individual-level change
(4) Structured curricula with clear and easy directions
(5) Consistent messages sent through multiple channels
(6) Emphasis on relationship building as a precursor to the delivery of program content
(7) Utilization of naturally occurring social networks and parental or social system involvement wherever possible
(8) Emphasis on integrating programs into clients real lives

(9) Strengths focus and asset rather than deficit modeling
(10) Continuity through high fidelity to the program, dosage adequacy, and consistency

Programs that include these components include LifeSkills Training (Botvin et al., 1990, 1995, 1997), Project ALERT (Ellikson, 1998; Ellikson, Bell, & McGuigan, 1993), and Project Northland (Pentz, Trebow, & Hansen, 1990).

A review of a few of these components can clearly demonstrate the need for cultural grounding. Component 1, for example, asks participants to incorporate life skills related to substance use into their behavioral repertoires. Geographical and cultural differences may make an understanding of certain substances more important or may render some skills more difficult to master. Refusal skills, for example, may be more difficult for a juvenile female of Korean descent where the importance of collectivity is strongly emphasized. Component 3 emphasizes community-building, a very different process depending on teens' cultural background. For instance, competent community building depends, to some extent, on the knowledge the practitioner has of how a particular ethnic community may work. Some groups are best approached through the elders or leaders of the community. Others might require that community building occur only the direction of a parent or an elder family member.

Component 9 involves helping the juvenile focus on strengths rather than deficits. Strengths and deficits may vary broadly depending on the experiences of particular communities or ethnic groups. As noted earlier, adolescents of Mexican descent living near the border often hold the traditions and customs of their ancestors more strongly than do others. This characteristic can be developed as a preventative strength, as it has been for Native-American youth in tribal prevention programming.

It is important to note that the SAMSHA model programs are abstinence-based. This has been a historical characteristic of prevention programs. As culturally grounded programs are developed, it may be important to reconsider this characteristic as well. Differential outcomes among juveniles who experiment with or use substances suggest that abstinence may be a useful approach for some while "harm-reduction" may be more effective for others. Differential characteristics of adolescents from other cultures may suggest this as well. One more obvious example is the Native-American youth involved with the Native-American Church who is faced with the choice of whether to use peyote as a part of the ceremonies.

Traditional HIV Prevention Models

Many promising HIV prevention programs have been developed for school settings. School-based prevention programs allow those who are actively involved in school to readily access services. They typically include a range of components such as education about HIV and risk behaviors, use of video and other media, demonstration of correct use of condoms, skill building through role plays, and discussion (Collins et. al., 2002). Participants have demonstrated significant increases in condom use (Blake et. al., 2003; Fisher, Fisher, Bryan, and Misovich, 1998; Kelly et al., 1991; St. Lawrence et al., 1995), decreases in the number of sexual partners (Jemmott, Jemmott, & Fong, 1992), and decreased sexual intercourse (Jemmott, Jemmott, & Fong; St. Lawrence et al.). Some have improved attitudes toward high-risk behavior (Fisher et al., 1998).

Community-based programs, offered at locations such as health clinics, churches, substance abuse treatment centers, and other community organizations (Amaro et al., 2001), attempt to reach youths who are irregular in their school attendance or do not attend school. Many emphasize HIV testing, condom use, safer sex negotiation skills, and self-efficacy for risk avoidance (Johnston et al., 2003). Community-based interventions have increased HIV knowledge and condom use among ethnic youth, homeless teens (Rotheram-Borus, Kooperman, Haignere, & Davies, 1991; Rotheram-Borus et al., 1997), gay and bisexual youth (Kelly et al. 1991; Rotherham-Borus, Reid, & Rosario, 1994), and youth in drug treatment (Joshi, Hser, Grella, & Houlton, 2001).

Effective prevention programs focus on reducing specific risk behaviors and are grounded in effective theoretical approaches. Effective strategies clearly communicate information about risks and stress avoidance of unsafe sexual behavior while consistently reinforcing healthy behavior. Many such programs also address peer pressure. Effective components include modeling new behaviors, practicing behavioral goal setting, and providing opportunities to practice negotiation and refusal. Participants also benefit from the use of diverse teaching methods that involve participants and allow them to personalize the curriculum. Programs are most effective when appropriate for participants' age, sexual experience, and culture. It is also critical that those leading the curriculum believe that it is valuable for participants (Kirby, 1999).

Identification of the components of successful and promising HIV prevention programs underscores the importance of cultural grounding in such programs. Being aware of the specific sexual behaviors that lead to infection within a given group allows practitioners to attend more thoroughly to those behaviors. Similarly, knowing whether specific techniques to protect against transmission (such as the use of condoms) are culturally encouraged or discouraged allows preventionists to tailor interventions to optimize the probability of use of the technique.

Culturally Grounded Substance Abuse and HIV Prevention

Little has been done to develop and evaluate programs for specific groups of adolescents such as those from ethnic minorities or in high-risk environments (Forgey, Schinke, & Cole, 1997). Most programs are created by and for European-Americans. Some have suggested that many program failures can be traced to their lack of cultural sensitivity (Hansen, Miller, & Leukefeld, 1995). The evidence offered in the current article supports this contention. Conversely, others have found that tailoring an intervention to a target population can increase its effectiveness (Marsiglia, Holleran, & Jackson, 2000). Such findings have led to a shift to culturally grounded programs (Botvin et al., 1995).

Although this shift is certainly desirable, it is also, almost certainly, inadequate. Referring again to the work of Silva (1983), differential conditions in the five life dimensions suggest that important differences exist where differential experiences have occurred. For example, in the dimension of life experience, the culture of students in traditional education programs varies dramatically from youth in general equivalency diploma (GED) programs, low-income community programs, and homeless shelters (Rew, Taylor, & Fitzgerald, 2001). Contextual factors including low socioeconomic status (SES), lack of school attendance, and lack of family stability have substantial influence on substance use (Freeman, 2001). Risk for school dropouts and homeless youth are compounded. Research shows that the rates of alcohol and other drug use are disproportionately high among both homeless and street youth (Greene, Ennett, & Ringwalt, 1997) as well as among delinquent youth generally (Barnes, Welte, & Hoffman, 2002).

Examining the overlap of ethnicity and alternative environmental cultures, Koopman and colleagues (1994) report that Hispanic homeless youth are more likely than are white or African-American juveniles to continue use of substances after leaving their home environments. However, a recent study conducted in an urban Texas community did not support this finding (Rew, Taylor-Seehafer, & Fitzgerald, 2001). These differential outcomes demonstrate the need for additional research into their implications for prevention interventions with high-risk youth. In addition, it is clear that culturally grounded research must consider not only cultural background but the diverse conditions that may exist in a juvenile's environmental context.

Some researchers consider the cultural adaptation of prevention programs unwise, citing the negative effect on intervention integrity. Castro, Barerra, and Martinez (2004) have responded, "While adaptation of prevention curricula is commonplace in agencies, prevention scientists still argue that fidelity outweighs the need for adaptation. However, awareness is growing that culturally adapted models are not only necessary, but the way of the future." Indeed, one must question the ethics of a decision to administer a "culturally neutral" intervention to groups for whom its effectiveness is likely to be diminished. The culturally neutral messages of universal substance abuse prevention programs ignore the unique strengths and needs of Mexican-American juveniles as well as other groups. Such programs are, in fact, based upon dominant culture and values: the behaviors and beliefs of Anglo, middle-class, male adults. As such, "neutral" messages enforce the dominant narrative, reflecting a view of the world that neither recognizes nor celebrates the minority child or the attendant minority cultural heritage. Culturally grounded prevention messages, on the other hand, aim to acknowledge and value community-based narratives as natural, indigenous prevention messages (Holleran, Reeves, Dustman, Marsiglia, 2002).

Toward Cultural Grounded Programs: The Drug Resistance Strategies Model

The Drug Resistance Strategies Project (DRS: R01 DA005629-08; 1997–2001) in Phoenix, Arizona, involved approximately 5,000 white, Latino, and African-American high-school youths from large city high schools in the creation of culturally grounded substance abuse prevention videos. The DRS followed previous research suggesting the utility of video-based approaches not only for engaging African-American and Latino youth but as an effective mode of intervention with these groups (Hecht, Corman, & Miller-Rassulo, 1993). The initial DRS project made the important contribution of combining core aspects of social influence models with the added integral component of cultural groundedness. The DRS study findings confirm the theoretical rationale for involvement of minority adolescents in the development of substance abuse prevention projects (Holleran, et al., 2002). The study utilized an experimental design incorporating videos as tools for depicting resistance strategies. The videos emphasized values and mores of varied cultures. For example, while the video depicting Anglo culture portrays individuality, independence from family, and identification with Anglo peers, the Latino video emphasizes familism, ethnic identifications with Latino peers and family, traditional Latino rituals, and language. Analyses of the DRS project data 14 months after intervention indicated (1) that students in the experimental schools had gained greater confidence in the ability to resist drugs, (2) increased use of the strategies taught by the curriculum to resist substance offers (control schools reported a decrease in the use of these resistance strategies), (3) more conservative norms adopted in both in school and at home, (4) reduction in the use of alcohol (a decrease of nearly 16% in the experimental group and an increase of slightly more than 20% in the control group), and (5) fewer positive attitudes toward drug use. The most striking implication for the proposed study, however, was that the curricula/videos that integrated elements of minority sociocultural norms were more successful with ethnic minority youth than the Anglo curricula/videos with significant effects on drug norms, attitudes, and use, particularly alcohol use. These findings support the importance of culturally grounded information in substance abuse prevention programs. Prevention messages that incorporate cultural elements and are presented within the social context of the participant are more likely to have a positive impact.

IMPLICATIONS FOR RESEARCH AND PRACTICE

The rationale, theory, and empirical results associated with culturally grounded prevention strongly argue in support of its implementation. This support has a number of implications for social work research and practice.

One important implication has to do with the inclusion of key components. The results produced by programs that include the SAMSHA-identified components have been positive for youth of the dominant culture as well as for several nondominant cultures. These components should be included when new programs are developed. Outcomes should consider the degree to which these programs are effective as well as whether differential outcomes exist when specific components are included or excluded.

It is also clear from rationale, theory, and research that, in order to optimize effectiveness, interventions must be adapted to consider cultural factors. Although the use of the key components is obviously important to intervention success, most can include culturally grounded modifications without threatening the integrity of the component itself. Videos and role-play, for example, can be augmented to include culturally relevant attitudes and perspectives. In such cases, the components themselves remain intact, yet their messages are packaged in a manner that will optimize the probability that they will be effective. Evaluators should consider whether integrity is genuinely affected. Where the components themselves are altered, evaluation techniques and conclusions must reflect this. Where they are not altered, researchers must refrain from allowing personal biases to impact their studies or, in fact, the programs themselves.

Just as cultural factors must be considered, adaptation for contextual factors is critical for intervention success. The examples offered earlier show the differential needs that exist between juveniles living in a more traditional home setting and those who are homeless or who are not attending school. Once again, in many cases these needs can be considered without doing violence to intervention integrity. When they cannot, the probability that intervention effectiveness will be enhanced should be weighed against the importance of integrity. When there is clear evidence from rational, theoretical, and empirical sources that intervention effectiveness is likely to be improved through adaptation for cultural or contextual factors, adaptations should be made. It is important to remember that evaluation exists to serve and inform intervention, not vice versa.

A fourth consideration identified in the earlier sections has to do with whether intervention goals should include abstinence, harm reduction, or some combination thereof. It is clear that what is appropriate for any group or any individuals within a group may not be appropriate for all groups or all members of any group. Acknowledgement of the high number of adolescents who report experimenting and even using substances regularly can lead to more realistic and effective prevention messages. Holleran, Taylor-Seehafer, Pomeroy, & Neff (in press) note that youth are not open to prevention efforts that they perceive are not "reality-based." The failure to acknowledge the aforementioned reality of youth experimentation and high rates of substance use undoubtedly would prohibit youth engagement with programming. Conversely, if substance use is realistically depicted in program and curriculum development, it is much more likely to resonate with the recipients and to have the desired impact. In fact, many prominent prevention scientists maintain that the key to effective prevention is the targeted audiences sense of ownership of the program (Price & Lorion, 1987; Kelly, 1987). This is not likely if they do not agree with the content and aims of the program.

The other important aspect of social work in the prevention realm are the concepts of "client centeredness" and "meeting the client where he/she is." While it is distasteful to accept that not only are many youth experimenting with substances, or using them sporadically or regularly, one must recognize that most youth who are at risk are not looking to abstain and may tune out vehement abstinence messages. Many adolescents have rejected or minimized prevention interventions, which touted drugs as "dangerous," "deadly," and "bad" in lieu of their own perceptions to the contrary.

One of the important considerations is that while abstinence may be the best intervention for those youth who are chemically predisposed for addiction or dependence, there is actually a continuum of youth between those who need abstinence and those who are considering use and those who are already using in small amounts to those who are in need of intervention. In the substance abuse and mental health field, there is awareness of the continuum of health care including universal, selective, indicated, case identification, standard treatment, long-term treatment, and aftercare (SAMSHA, 2002). Presently, universal prevention interventions focus only on the individuals who are not using in this continuum. There must be more attention paid to the gray areas between prevention and treatment. Harm Reduction Models serve as a bridge between these two erroneously dichotomized arenas.

Prevention programs for adolescents face many challenges because adolescents often do not perceive themselves to be at risk. They may view condom use negatively and often do not have the skills to negotiate safer sex practices. Topics covered in prevention programs, such as condom use and negotiating safer sex, are controversial in many communities. Improving the success of prevention programs will require addressing commonly held beliefs, including the idea that sex education will increase adolescent risk behavior (CDC, 2003a).

CONCLUSION

Traditional abstinence-based approaches to prevention provide an appropriate strategy for many individuals who are experiencing problems associated with substance use. This article provides an alternative perspective for work with those individuals for whom cultural or contextual factors may be critical, as well as those for whom abstinence may not be immediately appropriate.

For youths whose cultural background or contextual environment differs from that of the dominant culture, adaptation in curriculum to accommodate those differences can enhance intervention effectiveness. When used in conjunction with the this understanding of cultural and contextual influences, as well as the Stages of Change model, harm reduction and abstinence-based interventions can be seen as informing separate portions of the same continuum. An important skill in social work practice is determining the best fit when matching client needs with interventions. In some instances, harm reduction-based services potentially provide a better fit with clients' needs than the traditional abstinence-based interventions. In other instances, abstinence-based programming may be the appropriate choice.

Importantly, there does not appear to be an ethical dilemma created by the use of this perspective. In fact, it could be suggested that harm reduction actually provides a better fit than an abstinence-only perspective to social workers' mandates to maintain a commitment to clients' needs and to facilitate self-determination. As social workers become more familiar with perspective, it is hoped that other innovative interventions will be developed, both in work with individuals experiencing problems related to their substance use and in work with many other social problems.

REFERENCES

Alan Guttmacher Institute. (2002). Teenagers' sexual and reproductive health. In *Facts in Brief, January, 2002*. New York: Alan Guttmacher Institute. Retrieved November 1, 2003 from http://www.agi-usa.org

Amaro, H., Raj, A., Vega, R. R., Mangione, T. W., & Perez, L. N. (2001). Racial/ethnic disparities in the HIV and substance abuse epidemics: Communities responding to the need. *Public Health Reports, 116*, 434–448.

Archambault, D. L. (1992). Adolescence: A physiological, cultural, and psychological no man's land. In G. W. Lawson & A. W. Lawson (Eds.), *Adolescent substance abuse: Etiology, treatment & prevention*. Gaithersburg, MD: Aspen Publishers.

Atkinson, M., & Wing, S. (1998). *Counseling American minorities.* New York: McGraw Hill Publishers.

Bachman, J. G., Wadsworth, K. N., O'Malley, P. M., Johnston, L. D., & Schulenberg, J. E. (1997). *Smoking, drinking, and drug use in young adulthood: The impacts of new freedoms and new responsibilities.* Mahwah, NJ: Lawrence Erlbaum Associates.

Bandura, A. (1977). *Social learning theory.* Englewood Cliffs, NJ: Prentice Hall.

Barnes, G. M., Welte, J. W., & Hoffman, J. H. (2002). Relationship of alcohol use to delinquency and illicit drug use in adolescents: Gender, age, and racial/ethnic differences. *Journal of Drug Issues, 32*(1), 153–178.

Beauvais, F. (1992). An integrated model for prevention and treatment of drug abuse among American Indian youth. *Journal of Addictive Diseases, 11*, 63–80.

Beauvais, F. (1998). Cultural identification and substance use in North America: An annotated bibliography. *Substance Use and Misuse, 33*, 1315–1336.

Bhandari, S. (2004). *The survey of income and program participation: People with health insurance: A comparison of estimates from two surveys* (p. 243). Washington, DC: U.S. Department of Commerce, U.S. Census Bureau.

Blake, S. M., Ledsky, R., Goodenow, C., Sawyer, R., Lohrman, D., and Windsor, R. (2003). Condom availability programs in Massachusetts high schools: Relationships with condom use and sexual behavior. *American Journal of Public Health, 93*(6), 955–962.

Botvin, G. J., Baker, E., & Dusenbury, L. (1995). Long-term followup results of a randomized drug abuse prevention trial in a white middle class population. *Journal of the American Medical Association, 273*(14), 1106–1112.

Botvin, G. J., Baker, E., Dusenbury, L., Tortu, S., & Botvin, E. M. (1990). Preventing adolescent drug abuse through a multimodal cognitive-behavioral approach: Results of a 3-year study. *Journal of Consulting and Clinical Psychology, 58*(4), 437–446.

Botvin, G. J. (1997). Preventing adolescent cigarette smoking. *Journal of Developmental and Experimental Pediatrics 18*(1), 47–48.

Bukoski, W. J. (1985). School-based substance abuse prevention: A review of program research. In S. Ezekoye, K. H. Kumpfer, & W. J. Bukoski (Eds.), *Childhood and chemical abuse: Prevention and intervention.* NY: Hayworth Press.

Castro, F. G., Barrera, M., & Martinez, C. R. (2004). The cultural adaptation of prevention interventions: Resolving tensions between fidelity and fit. *Journal of Prevention Science 5*(1), 41–45.

Centers for Disease Control and Prevention. (2002). *Young people at risk: HIV/AIDS among America's youth.* Atlanta: U.S. Department of Health and Human Services, Centers for Disease Control and Prevention. Retrieved December 18, 2004, from http://www.cdc.gov/hiv

Centers for Disease Control and Prevention. (2003a). *HIV/AIDS surveillance report: Cases of HIV infection and AIDS in the United States, 2003* (pp. 1–9). Atlanta, GA: U.S. Department of Health and Human Services, Centers for Disease Control and Prevention. Retrieved December 18, 2004, from http://www.cdc.gov/hiv/stats/hasrlink.htm.

Centers for Disease Control and Prevention. (2003b). *National youth risk behavior survey: Trends in the prevalence of alcohol use.* Washington, DC: Author.

Centers for Disease Control and Prevention. (2003c). *Youth risk behavior surveillance 2003.* Atlanta: U.S. Department of Health and Human Services, Centers for Disease Control and Prevention. Retrieved December 17, 2004, from www.cdc.gov

Clayton, S. (1991). Gender differences in psychosocial determinants of adolescent smoking. *Journal of School Health, 61,* 115–120.

Collins, J., Robin, L., Wooley, S., Fenley, D., Hunt, P., Taylor, J., et al. (2002). Programs-that-work: CDC's guide to effective programs that reduce health-risk behavior of youth. *Journal of School Health, 72*(3), 93–99.

COSSMHO (National Coalition of Hispanic Health and Human Service Organizations). (1991). *HIV/AIDS—The impact on Hispanics in selected states.* Washington, D.C.: COSSMHO.

Eccles, J. S., & Barber, B. L. (1999). Student council, volunteering, basketball, or marching band: What kind of extracurricular involvement matters? *Journal of Adolescent Research 14,* 10–43.

Ellickson, P. L. (1998). Preventing adolescent substance abuse: Lessons from the Project ALERT program. In J. Crane (Ed.), *Social programs that work.* New York: Russell Sage Foundation.

Ellickson, P. L., Bell, R. M., & McGuigan, K. (1993). Preventing adolescent drug use: Long-term results of a junior high program. *American Journal of Public Health, 83*(6), 856–861.

Ellis, R. A., Klepper, T. D., & Sowers, K. M. (2000a). Similarity, diversity, and cultural sensitivity: Considerations for treating juveniles of African descent. *Journal for Juvenile Justice and Detention Services, 15*(1), 29–44.

Ellis, R. A., Klepper, T. D., & Sowers, K. M. (2000b). Building a foundation for effective intervention: Understanding Hispanic juveniles and their families. *Journal for Juvenile Justice and Detention Services, 15*(2), 26–39.

Falck, R., & Craig, R. (1988). Classroom-oriented, primary prevention programming for drug abuse. *Journal of Psychoactive Drugs, 20*(4), 403–408.

Finer, L. B., Darroch, J. E., & Singh, S. (1999). Sexual partnership patterns as a behavioral risk factor for sexually transmitted diseases. *Family Planning Perspectives, 31*(5), 228–236.

Fisher, J. D., Fisher, W. A., Bryan, A. D., & Misovich, S. J. (1998). Information-motivation-behavioral skills model based HIV risk behavior change intervention for inner city youth. *Health Psychology, 21*(2), 177–186.

Forgey, M. A., Schinke, S., & Cole, K. (1997). School-based interventions to prevent substance use among inner-city minority adolescents. In D. K. Willson, J. R. Rodrigue, & W. C. Taylor (Eds.), *Health-promoting and health-compromising behaviors among minority adolescents.* Washington, DC: American Psychological Association.

Freeman, E. M. (2001). *Substance abuse intervention, prevention, rehabilitation, and systems change strategies: helping individuals, families and groups to empower themselves.* New York: Columbia University Press.

Greene, J. M., Ennett, S. T., & Ringwalt, C. L. (1997). Substance use among runaway and homeless youth in three sample. *American Journal of Public Health, 87,* 229–235.

Guzman, B. (2001). The Hispanic population. Washington, DC: U.S. Census Bureau.

Hansen, W. B., Miller, T. W., & Leukefeld, C. G. (1995). Prevention research recommendations: Scientific integration for the 90's. *Drugs & Society, 8,* (3–4), 161–167.

Harmon, M. A. (1993). Reducing the risk of drug involvement among early adolescents: An evaluation of drug abuse resistance education (DARE). *Evaluation Review, 17,* 221–239.

Hecht, M. L., Corman, S., & Miller-Rassulo, M. (1993). An evaluation of the drug resistance project: A comparison of film versus live performance. *Health Communication, 5,* 75–88.

Holleran, L., Reeves, L., Marsiglia, F. F., & Dustman, P. (2002). Creating culturally-grounded videos for substance abuse prevention: A dual perspective on process. *Journal of Social Work Practice in the Addictions, 2*(1), 55–78.

Holleran, L. K., Taylor-Seehafer, M. A., Pomeroy, E. C., & Neff, J. A. (in press). Substance abuse prevention for high risk youth: Exploring culture and alcohol and drug use. In M. Delgado (Ed.), *Alcoholism Quarterly, special edition on Latinos and substance abuse.*

Jemmott, J., Jemmott, L., and Fong, G. (1992). Reductions in HIV risk associated sexual behaviors among black male adolescents: Effects of an AIDS prevention program. *American Journal of Public Health, 82*(3), 372–377.

Jessor, R. & Jessor, S. L. (1975). Adolescent development and the onset of drinking. *Journal of Studies on Alcohol, 36,* 27–51.

Jessor, R., & Jessor. S. L. (1977). *Problem behavior and psychosocial development. A longitudinal study of youth.* New York: Academic Press.

Johnston, L. D., O'Malley, P. M., & Bachman, J. G. (2003a). *Monitoring the Future national survey results on adolescent drug use: Overview of key findings, 2002* (NIH Publication No. 03-5374). Bethesda, MD: National Institute on Drug Abuse.

Johnston, L. D., O'Malley, P. M., & Bachman, J. G. (2003b). *Monitoring the Future national survey results on drug use, 1975–2002. Volume I: Secondary school students* (NIH Publication No. 03-5375). Bethesda, MD: National Institute on Drug Abuse.

Joshi, V., Hser, Y., Grella, C. E., and Houlton, R. (2001). Sex-related HIV risk reduction among adolescents in DATOS-A. *Journal of Adolescent Research, 16*(6), 642–660.

Kandel, D. B. (1982). Epidemiological and psychosocial perspectives on adolescent drug use. *Journal of American Academic Clinical Psychiatry, 21,* 328–347.

Kaplow, J. B., Curran, P. J., & Dodge, K. A. (2002). Child, parent, and peer predictors of early-onset substance use: A multisite longitudinal study. *Journal of Abnormal Child Psychology, 30*(3), 199–216.

Kelly, J. G. (1987). Seven criteria when conducting community-based prevention research: A research agenda and commentary. In J. A. Steinberg & M. M. Silverman (Eds.), *Preventing Mental Disorders: A Research Perspective* (DHHS Publication No. ADM 87-1492). Washington DC: U.S. Government Printing Office.

Kelly, J. A., St. Lawrence, J. S., Diaz, Y. E., Stevenson, L. Y., Hauth, A. C., Kalichman, S. C., et al. (1991). HIV risk behavior reduction following intervention with key opinion leaders of population: An experimental analysis. *American Journal of Public Health, 81*(2), 186–171.

Kirby, D. (1999). Reflections on two decades of research on teen sexual behavior and pregnancy. *Journal of School Health, 69*(3), 89–94.

Koopman, C., Rosario, M., Rotheram-Borus, M. J. (1994). Alcohol and drug use and sexual behaviors placing runaways at risk for HIV infection. *Addictive Behavior, 19*(1), 95–103.

Labouvie, E. (1996). Maturing out of substance use: Selection and self-correction. *Journal of Drug Issues, 26*, 457–476.

Lawson, G. W., & Lawson, A. W. (1992). *Adolescent substance abuse: Etiology treatment, and prevention.* Gaithersburg, MD: Aspen Publishers.

Lerner, J. V., & Vicary, J. R. (1984). Difficult temperament and drug use: Analysis from the New York longitudinal studies. *Journal of Drug Education, 14,* 1–8.

Lorion, R. (1987). Methodological challenges in prevention research. In D. Shaffer, I. Philips, & N. B. Enzer (Eds.), *Prevention of mental health disorders, alcohol and other drug use in children and adolescents.* OSAP Prevention Monograph-2. (DHHS Pub. No. ADM 90-1646). Washington, DC: U.S. Government Printing Office.

MacMaster, S. A., & Womack, B. G. (2002). Preventing HIV transmission among injection drug users: A brief history of syringe exchange programs *Journal of HIV/AIDS and Social Services, 1*, 95–112.

McQueen, A., Getz, J. G., & Bray, J. H. (2003). acculturation, substance use, and deviant behavior: Examining separation and family conflict as mediators. *Child Development 74*(6), 1737.

Marsiglia, F. F., Holleran, L., & Jackson, K. M. (2000). Assessing the effect of external resources on school-based substance abuse prevention programs. *Social Work in Education, 22*(3), 145–161.

McBride, N., Farringdon, F., & Midford, R. (2000). What harms do young Australians experience in alcohol-use situation? *Australian and New Zealand Journal of Public Health, 24*(1), 54–59.

McGuire, W. J. (1974). Communication-persuasion models for drug education: Experimental findings. In M. S. Goodstadt (Ed.), *Research on methods and programs of drug education.* Toronto: Addictions Research Foundation.

Neff, J. A., Crawford, S. L., and MacMaster, S. A. (2002). Ethnicity and multiple sex partners: An application of the health belief model. *Journal of HIV/AIDS & Social Services 3,* 41–65.

O'Donnell, L., O'Donnell, C. R., & Stueve, A. (2001). Early sexual initiation and subsequent sex-related risks among urban minority youth: The reach for health study, *Family Planning Perspectives, 33*(6), 268–275.

Pentz, M. A., Trebow, E. A., & Hansen, W. B. (1990). Effects of program implementation on adolescent drug use behavior: The Midwestern Prevention Program (MPP). *Evaluation Review, 14*(3), 264–289.

Price, R. H., & Lorion, R. P. (1987). Prevention programming as organizational reinvention: From research to implementation. In D. Shaffer, I. Philips, & N. B. Enzer (Eds.), *Prevention of mental health disorders, alcohol and other drug use in children and adolescents.* OSAP Prevention Monograph-2. (DHHS Pub. No. ADM 90-1646). Washington, DC: U.S. Government Printing Office.

Project DARE: How's it doing? (1990). Prevention File, 16-18. As cited in Harmon, M. A. (1993). Reducing the risk of drug involvement among early adolescents. *Evaluation Review, 17,* 221–239.

Ramirez, R. R., & de la Cruz, G. P. (2003). *The Hispanic Population in the United States: March 2002, Current Population Reports,* P20-545. Washington. DC: U.S. Census Bureau.

Rew, L., Taylor-Seehafer, M., & Fitzgerald, M. L. (2001). Sexual abuse, alcohol and other drug use, and suicidal behaviors in homeless adolescents. *Issues in Comprehensive Pediatric Nursing, 24*(4), 225–240.

Robins, L. N. (1980). The natural history of drug abuse. *Acta Psychiatrica Scandanavia, 62*(Suppl 284), 7–20.

Rotheram-Borus, M. J., Kooperman, C., Haignere, C., & Davies, M. (1991). Reducing HIV sexual risk behaviors among runaway adolescents. *JAMA: Journal of the American Medical Association, 266,* 1237–1241.

Rotheram-Borus, M. J., Reid, H., & Rosario, M. (1994). Factors mediating changes in sexual HIV risk behaviors among gay and bisexual adolescents. *American Journal of Public Health, 84*(12), 1938–1946.

Rotheram-Borus, M., Van Rossem, R., Gwadz, M., Koopman, C., & Lee, M. (1997). *Street Smart.* Retrieved December 18, 2004, from http://chipts.ucla.edu/interventions/manuals/intervstreetsmart.html

Savin-Williams, R. C., & Berndt, T. J. (1990). Friendship and peer relations. In S. S. Feldman & G. R. Elliott (Eds.), *At the threshold: The developing adolescent.* Cambridge, MA: Harvard University Press.

Scafidi, F. A., Field, T., & Prodromidis, M. (1997). Psychosocial stressors of drug-abusing disadvantaged adolescent mothers. *Adolescence, 32,* 93–100.

Segal, B., Cromer, F., Hobfoll, S., & Wasserman, P. Z. (1982). Reasons for alcohol use by detained and adjudicated juveniles. *Journal of Alcohol & Drug Education, 28,* 53–58.

Shedler, J., & Block, J. (1990). Adolescent drug use and psychological health: A longitudinal inquiry. *American Psychologist, 45,* 612–630.

Silva, J. S. (1983). Cross-cultural and cross-ethnic assessment. In C. Gibson (Ed.), *Our kingdom stands on brittle glass* (pp. 59–66). Silver Springs, MD: National Association of Social Workers.

Sly, D. F., Quadagno, D., Harrisson, D. F., Eberstein, I., & Riehman, K. (1997). The association between substance use, condom use and sexual risk among low-income women. *Family Planning Perspectives, 29*(3), 132–136.

St. Lawrence, J., Brasfield, T., Jefferson, K., Alleyne, E., O'Brannon, R., & Shirley, A. (1995). A cognitive-behavioral intervention to reduce African-American adolescents' risk for HIV infection. *Journal of Consulting and Clinical Psychology, 63*(2), 221–237.

Substance Abuse and Mental Health Services Administration (SAMHSA). (2002). *Science-based prevention programs and principles: Effective substance abuse and mental health programs for every community* (USDHHS publication number SMA 03-3764). Washington, DC: U.S. Government Printing Office.

Therrien, M., & Ramirez, R. R. (2000). *The Hispanic population of the United States.* Washington DC: U.S. Census Bureau.

Tobler, N. S. (1986). Meta-analysis of 143 adolescent drug prevention programs: Quantitative outcome results of program participants compared to a control comparison group. *Journal of Drug Issues, 4,* 537–567.

Tobler, N. S. (1989, October). Drug prevention programs can work: Research findings. Paper presented at the meeting of What Works: An International Perspective on Drug Abuse Treatment and Prevention Research, New York.

Tolan, P. H., Guerra, N. G., & Kendall, P. C. (1995). A developmental-ecological perspective on antisocial behavior in children and adolescents: Toward a unified risk and intervention framework. *Journal of Consulting and Clinical Psychology, 63,* 579–584.

U.S. Census Bureau, (2004). U.S. Interim Projections by Age, Sex, Race, and Hispanic Origin. Retrieved from the World Wide Web at http://www.census.gov/ipc/www.usinterimproj/>

U.S. Census Bureau (2002). Facts on the Hispanic or Latino Population. Retrieved from the World Wide Web at http://www.census.gov/pubinfo/www/NEWhispML1.html

Women in India: The Context and Impact of HIV/AIDS

Sonal R. Doshi
Bindi Gandhi

India is the second most populous country in the world. It is a young democracy that is dealing with all of the growing pains of being an emerging leader of the region and the world. The country has made strides in overcoming many of the obstacles related to developing a cohesive and working society in the nearly 60 years since independence. A major concern for India as a developing nation is its populations' health and well-being. In India, poor health outcomes are disproportionately affecting the economically disadvantaged (the lowest caste "Untouchables") and women (Menen-Sen & Shiva Kumar, 2001); women who are from lower castes face even more disadvantages and have even poorer health outcomes (Menen-Sen & Shiva Kumar). In addition, women are disproportionately affected by lack of employment opportunities, lack of educational access, and poor social status (Menen-Sen & Shiva Kumar). All of these conditions place Indian women at an extreme disadvantage when it comes to protecting themselves and their families against the HIV/AIDS epidemic that is spreading throughout India.

This article discusses women in India in the context of the HIV/AIDS epidemic and puts forth recommendations for a coordinated and cohesive response. To make these recommendations we discuss (1) the history of India; (2) India's population demographics, development, public health issues, and social norms regarding the treatment of women; (3) HIV/AIDS prevalence data and the most common routes of transmission; (4) the HIV/AIDS epidemic among women in India and how governments (local, state, and national) and various organizations have responded; and (5) three recommendations for tackling the epidemic among women in India.

BACKGROUND OF INDIA

India is described as living in "5 centuries at the same time" by Bollinger of Johns Hopkins, owing to the many apparent contradictions and diversity present in the country (Cohen, 2004: 508). In fact, an accurate description of India is hard to find as the country is constantly evolving (Cohen, 2004).

Historical Influences on the India of Today

India gained independence from Britain on August 15, 1947 under the leadership of Mohandas Gandhi. Gandhi focused attention on the plight of the "Untouchable" caste whom he renamed the Harijans, meaning "Children of God," some of whom belong to the Bhangi community. He also focused on education for all castes, meaningful employment, and public health issues such as sanitation and woman's rights and health (Gandhi, 1927). Within this context, the India the world knows today is actually quite young.

Caste and religious differences were defined and exploited both from those within the country (kings, the wealthy, etc.) and outside of the country (the British). The caste system has been used to segment Indian society into divisions based on birth (i.e., a person's caste is passed down from one generation to the next and may be changed only if a woman marries into a different caste, and even then, caste-based discrimination is still prevalent). The caste system also dictates the type of work a person is allowed to do (Bayly, 2001). Brahmans are allocated the task of religious and academic pursuits; they are the educators and temple priests and are many of the country's elected officials. The Bhangi community had been traditionally relegated to the task of removing human fecal waste. However, upon independence, the caste system was outlawed, and the Indian government made certain provisions in the Constitution for all of the castes that had a history of discrimination. These provisions included reserved spaces in the elected legislature, opportunities for government jobs, and education. The Indian government also made these same allocations for women. Though these structural changes were made to improve conditions for lower-caste members and women, social norms take much longer to change, and most members of Indian society still abide by these older norms, and discrimination continues. Members of these communities are often poor, consequently have low literacy levels, high infant mortality rates, and high rates of unemployment and poverty and, in today's environment, are victims of the HIV/AIDS epidemic.

India Today

India's population is spread over 28 states and 7 union territories. The national language is Hindi, which only 30% of Indians speak. There are an additional 14 official languages and hundreds of dialects that make communication very difficult; even the dialects can significantly differ from one another. The median age is less than 25 years, and a majority of the population is within the age range of 15–64 years (Central Intelligence Agency [CIA], 2005). Additionally, the majority of Indians (70%) live in rural areas (Government of India, 2001); however, the level of migration from rural to urban areas has been high owing to lack of employment opportunities and access to services in rural areas (Government of India, 2001). Twenty-five percent of India's population lives below the country poverty level, making India home to more than one-third of the world's poor (CIA, 2005; World Bank, 2004). Table 1 contains a summary of facts about India.

Unemployment is relatively low; however, the majority of poor families work in the informal sector (such as construction and house cleaning) wherein compensation is minimal and health risks are high (Thukral, 2002).

India's Development Status

The United Nations Human Development Index (HDI) is a means of measuring the different aspects of development for countries. The HDI for each country includes per capita consumption expenditure, incidence of poverty as captured by the head count ratio (the number of poor people as a proportion of total population), access to safe drinking water, proportion of households with *pucca* houses (permanent, not made from cardboard and corrugated metal), literacy rate for the age group 7 years and above, intensity of formal education, life expectancy at age 1, and infant mortality rates (Government of India, 2001). Government data show that the per capita expenditures on the different indices measured with the HDI have increased from the 1980s to the 1990s, with the level of spending (in $U.S.) in both urban and rural areas increasing. In the 1990s, there was more spent per capita in urban compared to rural areas in the following

TABLE 1. Summary Data on India

Area
  total: 3,287,590 sq km
  land: 2,973,190 sq km
  water: 314,400 sq km
  comparative—slightly more than one-third the size of the US
Population
  1,080,264,388 (July 2005 est.)
Age Structure
  0–14 years: 31.2%
  15–64 years: 63.9%
  >65 years: 4.9% (2005 est.)
Religion
  Hindu 80.5%, Muslim 13.4%, Christian 2.3%, Sikh 1.9%, other 1.8%, unspecified 0.1% (2001 census)
Median Age
  total: 24.66 years
  male: 24.64 years
  female: 24.67 years (2005 est.)
Population Growth Rate
  1.4% (2005 est.)
Birth Rate
  22.32 births/1,000 population (2005 est.)
Death Rate
  8.28 deaths/1,000 population (2005 est.)
Sex Ratio
  total population: 1.06 male(s)/female (2005 est.)
Infant Mortality
  total: 56.29 deaths/1,000 live births
  male: 56.86 deaths/1,000 live births
  female: 55.69 deaths/1,000 live births (2005 est.)
Life Expectancy at Birth
  total population: 64.35 years
  male: 63.57 years
  female: 65.16 years (2005 est.)
Total Fertility Rate
  2.78 children born/woman (2005 est.)
Literacy
  definition: > age 15 and can read/write
  total population: 59.5%
  male: 70.2%
  female: 48.3% (2003 est.)
Unemployment Rate
  9.2% (2004 est.)
Population Below Poverty Line
  25% (2002 estimate)

Note: From 2005 World Fact Book, by CIA, 2005, retrieved December 15, 2005, from http://www.cia.gov/cia/publications/factbook/print/in.html

categories: life expectancy ($3 vs. $2), formal education ($3 vs. $1.5), literacy ($3.75 vs. $2), *pucca* housing ($3.75 vs. $1.5), safe water ($4 vs. $2.5), and infant mortality ($2 vs. $1.25). The amount spent on poverty reduction in urban and rural areas was approximately the same at $1.25 per capital (Government of India, 2001).

Although some Indian states have made more progress in development and public health than others, there has been significant improvement in the entire country. The states having the highest ratings on the HDI are Kerala, Punjab, Tamil Nadu, Maharashtra, and Haryana. Not surprisingly, the states that have the lowest HDI are also the ones that are less economically developed, such as Andhra Pradesh and West Bengal (Government of India, 2001).

With a population of more than 1 billion people (CIA, 2005), resources to fund various government programs for targeted populations are scarce. Specifically, the fate of women in India is of major concern owing to this lack of resources and their status in Indian society. Females make up slightly less than one-half the population of India, a ratio of 1.06 males to 1 female. Women live slightly longer than do men (2 years longer) and have an average of 2.78 children (CIA, 2005). Of major concern is the fact that a little less than half the Indian female population is literate (CIA, 2005). Fewer girls than boys go to school, and the few who do go to school often drop out early (Menen-Sen & Shiva Kumar, 2001). The World Health Organization (WHO) reports that "a girl is 1.5 times less likely to be hospitalized than a boy and up to 50% more likely to die between her first and fifth birthdays" (WHO, 2005a: 26). In rural areas, Indian women have one of the highest maternal mortality rates in the world (Coonrod, 1998).

Public Health in India

The Indian Constitution requires the State to ensure health and nutritional well-being to all. Public health funding in India is scarce, although significant public health gains have been achieved since independence; death, birth, and infant mortality rates have significantly decreased while life expectancy has significantly increased in the past 50 years in urban and rural areas (Government of India, 2001). However, many issues still affect large sections of the population; women and children are extremely vulnerable to many of the causes of morbidity and mortality.

Every year, 1.2 million children die from diarrhea in India (Menon, 2004). Thousands more die of cholera, polio, hepatitis, worms, malaria, typhoid, and jaundice on an annual basis (Menon, 2004). Open defecation, common throughout the country, and poor solid waste management are the primary culprits. More than 80% of the diseases in India are attributable to unsafe drinking water (contaminants include fecal matter and chemicals) and improper sanitary practices. Every year, India deals with viral gastroenteritis, cholera, and typhoid epidemics— all preventable with access to clean water and efficient sewer systems. Of India's 300 major cities, about 70 have partial sewer systems and sewage treatment plants (Government of India, 2002). The bulk of untreated sewage ends up in India's rivers, lakes, and seas. Only 18—19% of homes in rural areas have toilets (Government of India, 2002). Since India's independence in 1947, political leaders have concentrated the country's limited financial resources on industry and science. Few financial resources have been allocated to basic public health infrastructure systems such as sewage systems; this leaves even fewer resources for addressing epidemics such as HIV/AIDS, let alone issues relevant specifically to women.

Women's Status in India

India's first prime minister, Jawaharlal Nehru, is quoted as saying, "You can tell the condition of a nation by looking at the status of its women." (Coonrod, 1998: first section). The role of women in Indian society has not quite progressed to the status of men. Discrimination against women in India can be divided into seven major areas: malnutrition, poor health, lack of education, overwork, lack of opportunity to obtain employable skills, mistreatment, and powerlessness. Women are often anemic and malnourished. Women from lower-caste groups face even more discrimination and health challenges. In urban hospitals, nurses in the labor ward often do not take the time to write patient case notes for women from lower castes, which deprives these women of safeguards given to other women of higher castes (WHO, 2005a). There are far fewer women in the workforce owing to lack of skills, and many of those who do work outside the home are underpaid and mistreated (Menen-Sen & Shiva Kumar, 2001). Violence, both in the home and outside of it, is not uncommon; every 26 minutes a woman is molested; rape occurs every 34 minutes; a woman is sexually harassed every 42 minutes; every 43 minutes a woman is kidnapped; and every 93 minutes a woman is killed (Menen-Sen & Shiva Kumar, 2001). Additionally, women often have the burden of household and community work. Women are under-represented in governance and decision-making positions. Women are legally discriminated against in property and land rights; they do not own property in their name and also do not inherit property (Menen-Sen & Shiva Kumar).

However, despite these statistics and information, India's constitutional laws regarding women can be considered progressive. India was one of the first countries in the world to give women the right to vote; the Indian constitution gives women some rights equal to those of men (Menen-Sen & Shiva Kumar, 2001). See Table 2 for the specific rights given to women in the Indian Constitution (Government of India, 2001).

In 1992, the National Commission for Women was established to safeguard the interests and rights of women by reviewing legislation that either directly or indirectly affects women. This Commission has focused on women from the Scheduled Castes and Scheduled Tribes (lowest castes, belonging to the Untouchable/Harijan castes) women/child-sex workers, women with disabilities, and women in similar vulnerable circumstances (Government of India, 2001). The Indian Government amended the following acts based on the Commis-

TABLE 2. Constitutional and Legislative Provisions for Women in India

The Constitution of India guarantees to all Indian women:

- Equality before the Law—Article 14;
- No discrimination by the State on grounds of only religion, race, caste, sex, place of birth or any of these—Article 15(1);
- Special provision to be made by the State in favour of women and children—Article 15(3);
- Equality of opportunity for all citizens in matters relating to employment or appointment to any office under the State—Article 16;
- State policy to be directed to securing for men and women equally, the right to an adequate means of livelihood—Article 39(a);
- Equal pay for equal work for both men and women—Article 39(d);
- Provisions to be made by the State for securing just and human conditions of work and for maternity relief—Article 42;
- To promote harmony and to renounce practices derogatory to the dignity of women—Article 51(A)(e).

In addition, Articles 243D(3), 243D(4), 243T(4) of the Constitution makes provision for reserving not less than one-third of the total seats for women in the direct elections to local bodies, viz. Panchayats (village elected officials) and municipalities.

Source: Government of India. National Human Development Report 2001. Planning Commission: New Delhi, 2001, p. 107. http://planningcommission.nic.in/reports/genrep/nhdrep/nhd2001.zip
Note: From National Human Development Report, by Government of India, 2001, p. 107. Retrieved December 15, 2005 from http://planningcommission.nic.in/reports/genrep/nhdrep/nhd2001.zip

sion's recommendations: The Commission of Sati (Prevention) Act of 1987, Immoral Traffic (Prevention) Act of 1956, Indecent Representation of Women (Prohibition) Act of 1986, Child Marriage Restraint Act of 1929, and many others related to rape, family, and guardianship (Government of India, 2001). This framework of legislation, rules, and procedures does not deter the violence and the violation of human rights that is still a common presence in the lives of many women in India. Regardless of the legal and judicial protections available to Indian women, the social norms and attitudes toward women have not kept pace with these advances. Also, the slow pace of justice and procedural requirements have eroded many of the legal safeguards for Indian women, making life very difficult (Government of India, 2001).

Social norms and attitudes have taken much longer to change and still do not match the changes in the Indian Constitution. Girls below the legal marriage age of 16 are often married off to older men. This is especially common in villages and in poor families where female children are married as quickly as possible so as to reduce household financial burden. Bigamy is still common and accepted. Married women are often deserted for other women or more commonly when the wife cannot bear children. If the wife is abandoned by her husband, she often has no place to turn to because her biological parents are no longer considered her family. In many villages, young, single women are promised high-paying jobs in the city that turn out to be work as commercial sex workers. Returning to their villages is not usually an option because of the stigma associated with the sex work they have engaged in or the debt they have accumulated and owe to their "employer." Many of these women also become HIV-positive (HIV+) and in turn could infect their potential offspring and other sexual partners.

Although gender inequality is still prevalent throughout the country, some states have done a better job than others of addressing the inequalities. The states of Kerala, Manipur, Mehalaya, Himachal Pradesh, and Nagaland have the highest levels of gender equality (Government of India, 2001). Overall, women are better off in southern India (Menen-Sen & Shiva Kumar, 2001). Kerala is often held as an example of gender equality, education and health outcomes, and access to services for women. Table 3 explains the "Kerala Model" and why Kerala as a state has been so successful in the area of women's rights (Jean & Sen, 1995).

There is a noted correlation between states that have improved female literacy levels and improvement in gender equality. It is im-

TABLE 3. Explaining the Kerala Experience

Kerala's success in social development, particularly given its relatively low level of per capita income, has attracted the attention of many development scholars both in India and abroad. The major factor behind the "miracle," according to a majority of scholars, is the remarkable expansion in literacy.

In 1998, Kerala reported a female literacy rate of 90%—significantly higher than the national average of 50% and comparable to many developed nations. Schooling is almost universal, with close to 97% of girls between 6–14 years attending school.

There are many other factors that have collectively contributed to Kerala's success.

- The massive educational expansion initiated by enlightened rulers in the pre-Independence era, further consolidated by State governments committed to health and education.

- The strong pro-poor and pro-people commitment of the left-leaning governments and of activist general politics.

- The adoption of redistributive measures, particularly land reforms.

- The widespread and equitable provision of health care and other public services.

- Several effective social reform movements that have contributed to ending traditional inequities.

- Enlightened public discussion leading to a cultural atmosphere that promotes greater freedom for women and a more active public role of women.

- A vigilant public aware of their rights and conscious of social justice.

Note: From India: Economic Development and Social Opportunity, by D. Jean & A. Sen, 1995.

portant to note that in the past few decades, gender disparities across Indian states have declined (Government of India, 2001). Interestingly, tribal societies in India tend to treat women better even though these societies are more illiterate and impoverished and have less access to resources (Menen-Sen & Shiva Kumar, 2001).

Women are more susceptible to HIV for a variety of biological and societal reasons. All of the foregoing characteristics and social attitudes make women all the more susceptible to HIV infection, especially from men. Dr. Peter Piot, Executive Director of UNAIDS, recently said, "The fight against HIV is tied to women's rights" (Girish, 2005).

HIV/AIDS in India

There are an estimated 5.7 million cases of HIV infection in India-the country with the highest number of HIV cases, exceeding South Africa for that dubious distinction (Joint United Nations Programme on HIV/AIDS [UNAIDS], 2006). The HIV/AIDS prevalence rate for India is 0.9%, with 5.7 million identified cases in a population of more than 1 billion people. India suffers from the "denominator problem"—the prevalence is low, but the raw numbers of Indians infected with HIV is high; the prevalence estimate is low because India's total population is so large. Based on this overall low prevalence rate, UNAIDS labels the country as a low prevalence country (UNAIDS, 2005a).

Of all cases of HIV infection among adults and children in India, 1.9 million cases are among women, and 0.12 million cases are among children (UNAIDS, 2004a).

Among all identified AIDS cases (individuals whose HIV infection has progressed to an AIDS-defining illness) as of July 2005, approximately 40% of cases are among females, ages 0-29 years old (National AIDS Control Organization [NACO], 2005a). Overall there is a 3:1 male-to-female ratio of total AIDS cases in India, and 87.7% of all AIDS cases are among the 15- to 44-year age group (NACO, 2005b).

Many professionals believe these estimates are very conservative and that the reality of the epidemic is much more alarming (Cohen, 2004; Sharma, 2000; U.N. official, 2005).

The epidemic in India is similar to that in Africa; it is primarily transmitted by heterosexual activity. This is in contrast to the epidemic in the United States wherein the gay male community and blood transfusion recipients were initially affected (Centers for Disease Control and Prevention [CDC], 1981, 1982). The primary modes of HIV transmission in India are heterosexual (85.7%), intravenous drug use (IDU) (2.2%), blood products/transfusion (2.6%), perinatal transmission (2.7%), and other (6.8%) (NACO, 2005b). Although the overall prevalence of HIV is less than 1%, the rates vary within states/regions of the country and among different subpopulations.

The National AIDS Control Organization has classified the states into high, moderate, and low prevalence (Table 4) (NACO, 2005b). These are classified based on the HIV/AIDS prevalence rate of pregnant women in antenatal clinics (ANCs)—the majority of the surveillance sites for the National HIV/AIDS prevalence estimation. The rates of infection among the subpopulations have been documented to vary nationwide. The rates of infection among IDUs are much higher in Manipur and the eastern states than in other states in India (NACO, 2005c). The same can be said for the rates among commercial sex workers (CSWs); their rates for HIV/AIDS infection are much higher in Maharashtra and Tamil Nadu than among a similar population in Bengal (NACO, 2005c). In the southern states of Tamil Nadu, Karnataka, and Andra Pradesh, the major mode of transmission is heterosexual contact with pockets of female CSWs being infected in

TABLE 4. Summary of HIV Prevalence Status among Indian States

High prevalence States[a]	Moderate prevalence States[b]	Low prevalence States[c]
Maharashtra	Gujarat	Remaining states and union territories
Tamil Nadu	Goa	
Manipur	Pondicherry	
Andhra Pradesh	• 4 districts in these states have been identified as high prevalence districts	
Karnataka		
Nagaland		
• 45 districts in these 6 states have been identified as high prevalence districts		

Based on consistent high prevalence of HIV as shown by HIV Sentinel data of last three rounds, 49 districts in the country have been identified as high prevalence districts for intensive program action.

Note: From An Overview of the Spread and Prevalence of HIV/AIDS in India, by National AIDS Control Organization, 2005. Retrieved December 15, 2005, from http://www.nacoonline.org/facts_overview.htm
[a]High prevalence states are cited as such because the HIV prevalence rates exceed 5% among high-risk groups and exceed 1% among antenatal women.
[b]Moderate prevalence states are cited as such because the HIV prevalence rates exceed 5% among high-risk groups but less than 1% among antenatal women.
[c]Low prevalence states are cited as such because the HIV prevalence rate is less than 5% in high risk groups, and less than 1% among antenatal women.

Maharashtra (NACO, 2005b, 2005c). In the past decade, HIV cases increased from 5,879 in 1991 to 5.1 million cases in 2003 (World Bank, 2003). In 2004, there was a sharp decline in the number of new infections from 520,000 in 2003 to 28,000 in 2004 (NACO, 2005d). Peter Piot, the Executive Director of the UNAIDS program, stated that "India having only 28,000 new infections is plainly impossible" (U.N. official, 2005). This sharp decline in new infections seems highly unlikely as many in the HIV/AIDS service community have not observed any change or increased the services they are offering (Solomon, Chakraborty, & Yepthomi, 2004). The non-governmental organization (NGO) Joint Action Council states that although the State AIDS Surveillance Centers send updated data to NACO, NACO's estimates remained unchanged (Sharma, 2000).

Many professionals believe these HIV prevalence estimates are very conservative and that the reality of the epidemic is much more alarming (Cohen, 2004; Sharma, 2000; U.N. official, 2005). These estimates may also be conservative because the majority of people in India do not know their HIV status. Confidential or anonymous HIV testing is not readily available nationwide, and the high level of social stigma and lack of confidentiality by the medical establishment discourages testing. Also, the infrastructure and policies for treatment and counseling services are not widespread or institutionalized (Godbole & Mehendale, 2005).

Surveillance is not conducted regularly at sites that individuals at risk for infection may frequent or among populations most at risk for HIV infection (e.g., IDUs, sexually transmitted disease [STD] patients, CSWs, and the like), and therefore the surveillance data have been very inconsistent over the years. In the early years of the epidemic, prior to the development of the National HIV Surveillance System by NACO in 1994, there was a strong sense of denial of the actual threat of HIV to India. The initial surveillance system was launched with only 55 sites in 3 of 32 states and union territories (World Bank, 2003). In 1998, the number of surveillance sites increased to 180. The number of sites increased to 232 sites in 2000 and to 670 sites in 2004 (NACO, 2005b). The initial surveillance sites were ANCs in predominantly urban areas and in 2000 sites targeting high-risk groups such as men who have sex with men (MSM) and CSWs were added to the surveillance program. In 2004, NACO started collecting data from 124 additional rural ANC sites, 166 STD sites, 13 IDU sites, 3 MSM sites, 2 CSW sites, 7 tuberculosis (TB) clinic sites, and 84 targeted intervention (TI) (CSW, MSM, and IDU) sites. Tuberculosis and TI sites were first monitored only in 2004 (NACO, 2005b). The addition of these extra sites will assist NACO in determining more representative prevalence estimates for the country.

In India, HIV/AIDS has also been expanding its reach to the rural parts of the country from major urban areas. There is concern that knowledge, awareness, prevention services, and treatment for HIV are scarce in many parts of the country although the disease has become more widespread (Godbole & Mehendale, 2005). Additionally, given the high levels of poverty and large population in rural areas, the tasks of outreach and service provision are daunting. Many researchers and activists warn that if India does not develop and implement a comprehensive prevention and treatment response to the HIV/AIDS epidemic in the near future, the epidemic is likely to follow the same pattern as Africa, with HIV heavily impacting all segments of society (Nagelkerke et al., 2002; United States National Intelligence Council, 2002).

Women and HIV/AIDS in India

Women account for approximately 40% of the HIV/AIDS prevalence in India. Women are increasingly more vulnerable to HIV infection because the major mode of transmission is heterosexual activity. There is growing evidence that the disease is spreading from high-risk populations into the general population with increasing rates seen at ANC sites (NACO, 2005c).

Infection rates among women and newborns are rising, owing to women's inability to protect themselves and negotiate for safer sex. There are many social precursors for the rapid spread of HIV in India, including the inability to talk openly and learn about sex and sexuality; pressures from family to give birth to an heir and an implicit threat to the marriage when a woman does not bear a child; the high prevalence and acceptability of domestic violence against women; the moral double standard imposed on men and women; and the lower status of women in general. The pressure to bear children is so intense that when a woman must choose between avoiding becoming infected with HIV by her husband but remaining childless or conception with the possibility of becoming HIV-infected, she often chooses the latter. As a result, three-fourths of HIV-positive women in India were infected within a few years of marriage (Solomon, Chakraborty, & Yepthomi, 2004).

Additionally, Indian women do not have ready access to condoms (male or female) or other means of protection. In many circumstances, Indian women also do not have the power to insist on the use of condoms with their partners (husbands or otherwise); this would imply that they themselves are unfaithful or that they do not trust their husband or partner, which may result in violence, abuse, or neglect (Go et al., 2003).

Because the first cases of HIV in India were identified among female CSWs, women in India have been blamed for the epidemic. Indian women are blamed although men constitute the majority of the cases (NACO, 2005b). However, in recent years more females are becoming infected than males as there are more women than males living with HIV in the 15- to 24-year age group (NACO, 2005a).

Voluntary counseling and testing (VCT) is not institutionalized in India; the obstacles of cultural and societal taboos on discussing sexuality and scarce treatment options are hard to surmount. This leads to little incentive for women to get tested. Many women who are aware of their husbands' HIV-positive status find little comfort at home; these women are at the mercy of the men in their families and often do not have the power or ability to protect themselves from becoming infected (Go et al., 2003). Many studies focusing on married, monogamous women in India document an increase in their rates of HIV infection (Divekar, Gogate, & Shivkar, 2000; Gangakhedkar et al., 1997; Mehendale, Shepherd, & Divekar, 1996; Rodrigues, Mehendale, & Shepherd, 1995; Ukey, Akulwar, & Powar, 2005). Studies have also found that the partners of these monogamous women are not faithful themselves, thus increasing these women's vulnerability to both STD and HIV infection (Ukey, Akulwar, & Powar, 2005). A recent prevalence study describes a decrease in the incidence of HIV among young women (15–24 years) attending ANC in four Southern Indian states from 2000 to 2004 (Kumar et al., 2006).

A significant association between STD infection and increasing risk for HIV infection has been described in the international data (Fleming & Wasserheit, 1999). There are very few large-scale/community-based studies of STDs and HIV in India. Smaller-scale, clinic-based studies in India have shown that genital ulcer disease and genital warts are significant risk factors for HIV infection (Risbud, 2005). Indian women are extremely vulnerable to STD infection for a number of reasons: biologically women are more susceptible than men to STDs; STDs are primarily asymptomatic in women and when symptoms do occur, they are usually not attributed to STDs; it is also more complicated to diagnose STDs in women. Additionally, male doctors in India are hesitant to do full physical exams (requiring touching their female patients' bodies) and take a sexual history because cultural taboos around this behavior are still prevalent.

The women in India who are at increased risk of becoming infected with HIV and those who are already infected are divided into three main categories for this discussion: commercial sex workers, wives of infected men, and pregnant women who are HIV-positive. The women in these categories have very specific characteristics and behaviors that need to be addressed in treatment and prevention programs.

Commercial Sex Workers

The history of the epidemic in India started with the first cases of HIV being detected in 1986 and 1987 in CSWs in Chennai, Madurai, and Vellore (John et al., 1987; Simoes et al., 1987). Commercial sex workers have always been regarded with stereotypes and mistrust in India and worldwide. Many of the CSWs in India who are in the major cities congregate in red-light districts. The CSWs in India generally have little power over their work environment and even their own clients; they are in many cases indentured to their madams or pimps and do not have the power to negotiate condom use or other means of safer sex with their clients. These girls and women are extremely vulnerable to exploitation. Many have little or no formal education. Many female CSWs are infected with STDs, and this infection makes them more susceptible to HIV infection (Hawkes & Santhya, 2002; Risbud, 2005).

HIV rates among female CSWs have been extremely high since cases were first identified. Most of the data collected for this population over the years has been through small-scale studies. NACO has only recently added CSW sites as part of their national Surveillance Program sites. There are presently two sites officially collecting HIV surveillance data for this population (since 2001; NACO, 2005b). The rates among CSWs in Mumbai range from 58.7% (2000) to 44.7% (2004; NACO, 2005c). In smaller studies, rates range from 2.5% to 69% in Mumbai, 34% to 54% in Pune, and 43.2% in Surat (Godbole & Mehendale, 2005).

Wives and Partners of HIV-Infected Men

A primary HIV prevention message has been that if one is monogamous and uses condoms, one will be able to protect oneself from infection by HIV and other STDs. Increasingly, numbers of Indian women are discovering that although they adhere to the values and cultural norms of monogamy and marriage, their husbands or partners may not, resulting in increasing numbers of STD infections, including HIV among married and monogamous women in India (Gangakhedkar et al., 1997; Ukey, Akulwar, & Powar, 2005).

The lack of power Indian women have in many of their relationships (with husbands, in-laws, and community) has put them at the mercy of the men around them. In this culture, it has been difficult for women to be assertive and protect themselves from HIV infection. Service providers are educating women about their rights and about using condoms as a method of protection. Women, especially women with HIV, are economically and sexually vulnerable to their husbands. They are often at the mercy of their husbands for financial support, expected to fulfill traditional family roles, and are often accused of bringing shame to their family even if it was the actions of their husband that brought this "shame."

Transmission of HIV among couples in India has been documented in the past decade and a half. Data have shown that women attending STD clinics who were not CSWs had a prevalence of HIV infection of 13.6%, with a majority of these women reporting only one sexual partner (their husband; Gangakhedkar et al., 1997). In another study, wives of IDUs in Manipur were shown to be at a higher risk of HIV infection (45% of HIV+ IDU users' wives were HIV+) (Panda et al., 2000). Studies that have examined the prevalence of HIV infection in married women have found that their husbands' reported behavior was the major risk factor for many of these women.

A study of long-distance truck drivers in South India showed that 74% of the HIV+ drivers were married, 38.7% of study participants had an STD of some sort, and overall 86% of these men had extramarital sex. The men who had extramarital sex were also significantly more likely to have sexual contact with CSWs, have multiple sexual partners, and have an HIV+ diagnosis than were men who remained faithful to their wives/partners (Manjunath, Thappa, & Jaisankar, 2002).

Another study of MSM activity among rural Indian men showed that 10% of single men and 3% of married men had unprotected anal sex with a man in the past year. The married men who reported MSM activity were also more likely to report sex with their wives and other female partners over the year. Eleven percent of this population also reported anal sex with their female partners (Verma & Collumbien, 2004).

In contrast, a recent prevalence study has described a decrease in the HIV-1 incidence among young women (15–24 years) attending ANCs in four South Indian states from a rate of 1.7% in 2000 to 1.1% in 2004. This is a relative reduction of 35%, which is promising though there were not similar decreases seen for women in the older age groups or women in other parts of the country (Kumar et al., 2006).

Pregnant Women and their Children

Pregnant women who are HIV+ are also criticized and ostracized. They may likely not have access to antiretroviral (ARV) therapy and may deliver an HIV+ child (Merchant & Lala, 2005). With intensive ARV therapy, the risk drops from 30% to 45% to 2% risk that their children will be born infected (Merchant & Lala, 2005). Very few women in India have access to antenatal care or assistance during delivery to ensure a safe delivery let alone treatment for prevention of mother-to-child-transmission (PMTCT). Data show that only 65% of pregnant women receive one or more prenatal visits and only 30% received more than four visits. Additionally, only 43% of births are attended by skilled health personnel, and only 34% of deliveries are in health facilities (WHO, 2005a)—a consequence of the fact that the majority of Indians live in rural areas. The health care infrastructure and resources allotted to women's health issues is scarce; women who live in rural areas have even less access to health care and rarely have access to basic services such as hospitals and clinics (WHO, 2005a).

For appropriate treatment to take place, the women have to know their status and deliver in facilities where treatment options are available. In India, it is customary for women to go to their own parents' home at the time of delivery. This further complicates continuity of care and services as they often live far from their parents' home and will see a different health care provider than the one they had been seeing for prenatal treatment. Many women use traditional midwives for delivery, and their knowledge of prevention and treatment options maybe limited.

Not only are pregnant women vulnerable, their children and families may also be victims of this deadly disease. If the newborn is infected, access to medications for mother and baby are not easily accessible (financially or otherwise) in India (Merchant & Lala, 2005). Additionally, if the mother or baby is discovered to be HIV+, there are many family, personal, and societal repercussions. A devastating situation for all is when the women and children are ostracized and left to their own scarce resources.

The rates of HIV infection among pregnant women have increased in some parts of the country based on surveillance data (Andra Pradesh went from 1.5% in 2000 to 2.25% in 2004; Delhi went from 0.25% to 0.38%; Madhya Pradesh went from 0.12% to 0.25%; Manipur went from 0.75% to 1.5%; and Nagaland from 1.35% to 1.43%). Other areas wherein rates are greater than 1.0% are Goa, Karnataka, Maharashtra, Mumbai, and Mizoram (NACO, 2005c). The seropositivity rate among pregnant women in selected sentinel sites ranges between zero and a high of 8.75% in Churachandpur (UNAIDS, 2004b).

INDIA'S RESPONSE: WOMEN AND HIV/AIDS

India is a country that has limited resources and is struggling with many infrastructure, economic, and health concerns for its citizens. In 2002, the Indian government spent only 6.1% of its gross domestic product (GDP) on health expenditures; a steady increase from the 5.2% spent in 1998 (WHO, 2005). The 2002 per capita government expenditure on health averaged US$6 while the overall per capita total health expenditure (per capita combined total of government and private expenditure on health) was US$30 (WHO, 2005).

The government has been very careful about how money is allotted and have focused its resources on program areas where there has been shown to be high rates of success and which affect large populations. It is with this mindset that India has focused on water-borne diseases; public health infrastructure such as access to clean water and sewage systems; treatable health problems such as TB, anemia, and malnutrition; and basic rights such as education. Though India is extremely large in both mass and population and these issues seem overwhelming at times, it must be remembered that public health problems are interrelated and that the women who do not have access to education may become CSWs to financially support themselves and their families; the women who are diagnosed with pneumonia or TB may also have HIV; and the cycle continues. Bill Gates stated, "The choice now is clear and stark: India can either be the home of the world's largest and most devastating AIDS epidemic—or, with the support of the rest of the world, it can become the best example of how this virus can be defeated" (Gates, 2002). There are many who believe that India should first deal with basic health issues such as malaria and malnutrition before addressing the HIV/AIDS epidemic, as there is no known cure, the treatment medications are very expensive, and frank discussions around sexual behavior and protection are not "culturally appropriate." These two messages are diametrically opposed and so the question remains: What should India do to deal with this epidemic?

At the time that HIV was infiltrating the population in the mid-1980s, the country was struggling with a sparse public health and medical infrastructure to deal with a plethora of health conditions, with HIV and AIDS being yet another problem to deal with. The government was slow to initially respond to the epidemic because of denial that the disease had really made its way to India. The initial victims were CSWs and IDUs (John, Babu, Jayakumari, & Simoes, 1987; Simoes et al., 1987), already marginalized populations which did not encourage the government to respond quickly.

The primary players in the response to the HIV epidemic in India are the central and state governments of India, the international donor community, and NGOs. The main body within the central Indian government that is coordinating the response to the epidemic is the NACO that was established in the Ministry of Health and Family Welfare. The program's main activity at the start of the epidemic was monitoring HIV infection rates in select urban areas. The government's strategy then changed in 1991 to implement initiatives such as HIV testing centers, strengthening blood safety, and controlling hospital infection in addition to taking over surveillance activity from the Indian Council of Medical Research (ICMR). There are now NACO centers in all the state capitals of India in addition to the major cities (NACO, 2005b).

NACO's role has been to implement the programs set forth by the National AIDS Control Project (NACP). These programs have been rolled out in "phases." The first phase focused on initiating a national commitment, increasing awareness, and addressing blood safety issues. Some of these objectives were achieved, such as increased awareness and changes in blood donation processes; professional blood donations were banned by law, and screening of donated blood became more standard practice. There were variations in performance by state and region of the country. The bulk of the funding for this phase of the project came from an $84 million International Development Association (IDA) credit supplemented by World Health Organization/Global Program on AIDS (WHO/GPA) co-financing of $2.2 million and an Indian government contribution of $27.5 million (World Bank, 2003).

India is now in the second phase. The government is continuing to expand programs at the state level, and there is a stronger emphasis on targeted interventions for high-risk groups (i.e., CSWs, truck drivers, IDUs, migrant laborers, and MSM) and prevention initiatives among the general population. There is continued support for involving NGOs and other governmental departments (education, transportation, and police) in the implementation of programs. There is also to be a stronger focus on monitoring and evaluating the projects being implemented, which may lead to more targeted programming for women with HIV and at risk of becoming infected with HIV. The government is now in the planning stages for phase three of the NACP. It is expected that this process will include nationwide consultations with national stakeholders in addition to international development partners. The Indian government is expected to expend $45 million of its own funds for phase two (World Bank, 2003).

Other government supported programs include networks of people living with HIV/AIDS, 722 VCT centers as of December 2004, support of HIV/AIDS programming on Doordarshan (government-sponsored broadcaster), phase 1 clinical trial for an HIV vaccine, and in 2004 the government started providing free ARV therapy to people living with HIV/AIDS at government hospitals in six high-prevalence states and the city of Delhi (NACO, 2004a). Also 2004 brought a change in government; the Bharat Janata Party (BJP) was voted out of office. During their tenure in the government, the BJP focused on health, though they seemed to purposefully stay away from addressing the HIV/AIDS issue. In 2004, the Congress party was voted back into government after being out of power for many years. The Congress party has increased political commitment to implement a program on HIV and AIDS involving all public and private sectors (UNAIDS, 2005b).

There has been a heavy reliance on NGOs and international development donors to assist with the response to the epidemic in India. The NGOs have raised awareness and reached high-risk groups. Although NGOs in India have been involved in health, family planning, and other development issues for years, very few NGOs had experience in the design and implementation of HIV/AIDS activities/programs. They also did not have experience with the populations at highest risk for HIV infection (CSWs, IDUs, or MSM). Presently there are numerous NGOs working on HIV/AIDS issues at the local, state, and national levels (NACO, 2005e). They are involved in interventions with high-risk groups, direct care, general awareness campaigns, working with AIDS orphans, and the like. Funding for these NGOs come from a variety of sources such as the federal or state governments of India, local contributors, and international donors.

There are a large number of international donors working in India or funding programs/projects in India. Many UN agencies (UNAIDS, WHO, United Nations Children's Fund, United Nations Development Programme, United Nations Population Fund, and others) provide technical assistance and other support through their country offices and partnerships in India. These collaborations have been in place since the early 1990s if not before. Also, there has been much financial and technical support from the United Kingdom Department for International Development, Canadian International Development Agency, Australia, the United States (USAID and CDC), and funding through the Global Fund (NACO, 2004b). Additionally, the Global Fund has funded programs for PMTCT and TB/HIV co-infection, the Gates Foundation has pledged a tremendous amount of money through the Avahan Initiative, and the World Bank continues to be a main financier for the Indian government's programs.

Prevention messages have also been embedded in the media outlets, from popular Bollywood films to radio soap operas (Population Communications International, 2005). The Bollywood films "Phir Milenge" and "My Brother Nikhil" focus on individuals who are

HIV+ and then face discrimination by society. However, both of these films fall short of addressing the audiences who currently have the highest prevalence rates: truck drivers, sex workers, and spouses of both of these populations.

The result of much of the programming has shown the importance of locally focused and targeted messages and the need for programs to incorporate local languages, cultural norms, address caste issues, and societal issues in regard to sex, and so on. This all makes working within the context of an Indian community very difficult and highlights the fact that there will not be one solution for every situation. Large gaps in access to basic services for women in India need to be addressed in tandem with the more targeted approach of education and treatment. The improvement in the basic services for women will ensure that programs have the potential to succeed and develop long-term sustainability.

The attempt at a comprehensive approach to improving life for women in India has been reflected in government programs, legislation, and the many programs that national NGOs have been implementing (Freedom Foundation in Bangalore, Lawyers Collective, MILANA-Action AID, and other NGOs; NACO, 2005e). Both government and NGOs have been somewhat successful in establishing policy and programs targeted at women and bridging the economic, health, and social gap with their Indian male counterparts. Successful NGO programs have focused on improving literacy among specific female populations with low literacy rates (rural women, women from lower castes, and women in high-risk groups), providing alternative forms of employment (encouraging use of traditional art and embroidery) while increasing compensation, nutrition supplements, and health education (United States Agency for International Development [USAID], 2005). For example, the Self Employed Women's Association (SEWA) was created to target marginalized poor women in both urban and rural areas; SEWA utilizes a multi-pronged approach to working on women's issues-employment options, skills building, literacy classes, health education classes, nutrition supplements, a micro-loan program, and a variety of programs to encourage self-confidence and empowerment in a population without access to these options (SEWA, 2005).

Several NGOs have also created very successful programs that have increased awareness of HIV/AIDS as an important public health issue and have created behavior change among high-risk populations such as sex workers and truck drivers (Family Health International, 2000;

Jana, Basu, Rotheram-Borus, & Newman, 2004). These programs are very grassroots and tend to employ and use community members as peer educators for the targeted community.

There have been some successful attempts to specifically assist women to empower themselves to protect themselves from STDs and HIV infection. Sonagachi is a prime example of a program targeted specifically at CSWs to empower them; it includes health clinics and sex workers who are hired as peer educators for peer outreach. Another aspect of the program is that the women have set up their own bank so as not to have to deal with loan sharks. The program is lauded as a "Model effort by WHO." A small-scale replication project was done in two other sex worker communities in West Bengal, showing an increase in condom use that was sustained over 16 months (Basu et al., 2004). See Table 5 for additional information on the Sonagachi Project.

TABLE 5. Case Study: Sonagachi Project

Sonagachi is the largest red light district in Calcutta and the Sonagachi Project was started in 1992 primarily to assess the prevalence of STDs and HIV among the sex workers. This project was the brainchild of Smarajit Jana.

The Sonagachi Project is so successful primarily because it responds to the community's needs by creating an enabling environment allowing the sex workers to target their own community on their own behalf; they were recognized as the change makers in the community. Additionally, the project did not judge the sex workers, instead the sex workers were accepted for who they are, the lifestyle in which they live, and their range of emotional and material needs. The sex workers themselves designed the program activities and actively participated in every level of the program planning. Many experts agree (Basu et al., 2004) that another reason this project was so successful is because there was support for this project by highly influential community and government leaders who have political and social clout.

The intervention project consists of three components: providing health services including STD treatment from a central clinic in the area; dissemination of IEC messages regarding prevention of STD/HIV transmission; and promotion of condom use. Sonagachi sex workers are the peer educators used for the health education outreach.

Program Successes:

• Genital ulcer has reduced from 6.22% in 1992 to 0.99%.

• HIV prevalence has remained stable within 5% during 1995 to 1998, which is remarkably low for this community.

• Condom use has increased from 2.7% in 1992 to 80.5% in 1998.

Several other organizations are attempting to replicate Sonagachi's success—Saheli in Pune is attempting to create the project with their sex worker group.

Note: From Creating an enabling environment: Lessons learnt from the Sonagachi Project, India, by S. Jana, N. Bandyopadhyay, A. Saha, & M. K. Dutta, 1999, *Research for Sex Work*, 2, 22–24.

RECOMMENDATIONS

If India does not do anything more about the issue of HIV/AIDS, for women especially, the country may face an epidemic of major proportions; infection rates may continue to soar and possibly at much higher rates. Some researchers have estimated that India could have up to 25 million HIV cases by 2010 (Nagelkerke et al., 2002; United States National Intelligence Council, 2002). Even with current reported data, the prevalence rate reported is only the tip of the iceberg. Most experts believe that there are many more infections than reported by surveillance data (Zaheer, 2005). The HIV situation in India may not have been alarming at first glance; however, a small percentage-point rise in HIV incidence must be viewed in absolute numbers as well as a proportion of a billion or more inhabitants. There are new data describing a decrease in HIV incidence among young women attending ANCs in four south Indian states; this is very promising news. It is still extremely important that a focus is maintained to develop a cohesive and broad-based prevention and treatment program for India. These data are applicable only to a small population of women in the country (rates in the northern states did not vary significantly from 2000 to 2004) and also do not address the rates among CSWs (Kumar et al., 2006).

India's approach for attacking HIV and AIDS among its female population should be multi-pronged and multi-leveled for most effectiveness. The Indian government and international NGOs need to work more closely with partners at the grass-roots level in order to ensure program effectiveness and success. This means ensuring that all program planning and implementation occur with the complete involvement of the communities in question and take into account local languages and norms. There also should be inclusion of all members of the community in the planning and implementation of programs and messages to be disseminated. Mothers, fathers, husbands, brothers, sisters, children, religious leaders, and medical personnel all need to be involved in prevention, education, treatment, and the de-stigmatization of HIV/AIDS.

India should focus on short-term, intermediate, and long-term solutions to deal with this situation. The short-term solutions should focus on providing more access to treatment and care for women with HIV because it is these women who are potentially infecting their fetuses, sharing bodily fluids with men who purchase sexual acts for money, and are not able to care for themselves, let alone their children. The benefits of these programs will be seen in 1–5 years (Dandona,

2002). The intermediate solutions should include more education and skill building around HIV for women, men, and children, and more access to HIV testing, condoms and other female-controlled measures (female condom, vaginal microbicides) to prevent HIV. The benefits of focusing on HIV education will be seen in 5 to 10 years.

India's long-term solutions should include a focus on broader changes in the context in which women live: access to education for all girls, including higher education; alternative employment options for women so that they are not dependent upon their husbands for financial security (this must be done in a culturally sensitive manner); improve the overall health of women and children by lowering the maternal and infant mortality rates; increase access to nutritional foods to alleviate anemia and malnutrition; provide more opportunities for women to be included in decision-making roles in local, state, and country government (the Constitution has certain allotments for women but they are not being filled—more ground and grassroots work should be done around this issue); and finally, encourage the change of cultural and attitudinal norms within the larger sphere of Indian society so that men do not feel that it is socially acceptable to beat, rape, or hurt their wives and for the overall society to view and treat women with the respect and dignity that they are due. India needs to focus on all three types of solutions for positive results to be achieved in addressing HIV/AIDS and women's health and social welfare. These three programmatic areas are inherently linked to each other and by working on all prongs of the plan, there is likely to be a more sustained impact and improvement of life for everyone on the Indian subcontinent.

Although it is true that there are many challenges involved in expanding the high-level commitment to all states and to the grass-roots level, as well as in involving ministries and departments other than health, and in scaling up interventions to meet the projected needs for prevention and care, "India's socioeconomic status, traditional social norms, cultural myths on sex and sexuality, large-scale migration and a huge population of marginalized people make it extremely vulnerable to the AIDS epidemic" (UNAIDS, 2005, top of section).

> *"That future is not one of ease or resting but of incessant striving so that we may fulfill the pledges we have so often taken and the one we shall take today . . ."*

> *"The future beckons to us. Whither do we go and what shall be our endeavour? To bring freedom and opportunity to the*

common man, to the peasants and workers of India; to fight and end poverty and ignorance and disease; to build up a prosperous, democratic and progressive nation, and to create social, economic and political institutions which will ensure justice and fullness of life to every man and woman."

(Jawaharlal Nehru, "Tryst with Destiny."Address to the Constituent Assembly. New Delhi, August 14 and 15, 1947. Reprinted from Government of India. *National Human Development Report*, 2001, 2.)

REFERENCES

Bayly, S. (2001). *Caste, society and politics in India from the eighteenth century to the modern age*. New York: Cambridge University Press.

Basu, I., Jana, S., Rotheram-Borus, M. J., Swendeman D., Lee, S., Newman, P., et al. (2004). HIV prevention among sex workers in India [Electronic version]. *Journal of the Acquired Immune Deficiency Syndrome, 36*, 845–852.

Centers for Disease Control and Prevention. (1981). Pneumocystis pneumonia—Los Angeles. *Morbidity and Mortality Weekly Report, 30*(21), 1–3.

Centers for Disease Control and Prevention. (1982). Current trends update on acquired immune deficiency syndrome (AIDS)—United States. *Morbidity and Mortality Weekly Report, 31*(37), 507–508, 513–514.

Central Intelligence Agency. (2005). *World Fact Book 2005*. Retrieved December 15, 2005, from http://www.cia.gov/cia/publications/factbook/geos/in.html

Cohen, J. (2004). HIV/AIDS: India's many epidemics [Electronic version]. *Science, 304*, 504–509.

Coonrod, C. (1998). *Chronic hunger and the status of women in India*. Retrieved December 12, 2005, from http://www.thp.org/reports/indiawom.htm

Dandona, L. (2002). HIV/AIDS control in India [Electronic version]. *Lancet, 360*, 1789.

Divekar, A. A., Gogate, A. S., & Shivkar, L. K. (2000). Disease prevalence in women attending the STD clinic in Mumbai (formerly Bombay), India. *International Journal of STD & AIDS, 11*, 45–48.

Family Health International. (2000). *Prevalence of sexually transmitted infections and HIV among long distance inter-city truck drivers and helpers of Northern India*. Retrieved December 16, 2005, from http://www.fhi.org/NR/rdonlyres/epyfmkvc5ppf5tzy4s7m4ddynf7w4mzkujegzd4hvckjtidvdofvbu6qiih2y7kkwxjjif w2ht7rbl/PrevalenceofSexuallyTransm.pdf

Fleming, D. T., & Wasserheit, J. N. (1999). From epidemiological synergy to public health policy and practice: the contribution of other sexually transmitted diseases to sexual transmission of HIV infection. *Sexually Transmitted Infections, 75*, 3–17.

Gandhi, M. (1927). *Gandhi an autobiography: My experiments with truth.* Ahmedabad, India: Navajivan Trust.

Gangakhedkar, R. R., Bentley, M. E., Divekar, A. D., Gadkari, D., Mehendale, S. M., Shepherd, M. E., et al. (1997). Spread of HIV infection in married monogamous women in India [Electronic version]. *Journal of the American Medical Association, 278,* 2090–2092.

Gates, B. Slowing the spread of AIDS in India. *New York Times.* Retrieved December 12, 2005, from http://law.gsu.edu/ccunningham/fall02/NYTimes-Nov9-AIDSinIndia-ByBillGates.htm

Girish, M. (2005). The disease of being a woman. *Indian Express.* Retrieved November 18, 2005, from www.indianexpress.com

Go, V. F., Sethulakshmi, C. J., Bentley, M. E., Sivaram, S., Srikrishnan, A. K., Solomon, S., et al. (2003). When HIV-prevention messages and gender norms clash: The impact of domestic violence on women's HIV risk in slums of Chennai, India. *AIDS Behavior, 7*(3), 263–272.

Godbole, S., & Mehendale, S. (2005). HIV/AIDS epidemic in India: Risk factors, risk behaviour & strategies for prevention & control [Electronic version]. *Indian Journal of Medical Research, 121,* 356–368.

Government of India. (2001). *National Human Development Report.* New Delhi: Planning Commission, Government of India. Retrieved December 1, 2005, from http://www.planningcommission.nic.in/reports/genrep/nhdrep/nhd2001.zip

Government of India. (2002). *India assessment 2002—water supply & sanitation.* New Delhi: Planning Commission, Government of India, 2002. Retrieved April 3, 2006 from http://planningcommission.nic.in/reports/genrep/wtrsani.pdf

Hawkes, S., & Santhya, K. G. (2002). Diverse realities: Sexually transmitted infections and HIV in India [Electronic version]. *Sexually Transmitted Infections, 78,* 31–39.

Jana, S., Bandyopadhyay, N., Saha, A., & Dutta, M. K. (1999). Creating an enabling environment: Lessons learnt from the Sonagachi Project, India [Electronic version]. *Research for Sex Work, 2,* 22–24.

Jana, S., Basu, I., Rotheram-Borus, M. J., & Newman, P. A. (2004). The Sonagachi project: A sustainable community intervention program [Electronic version]. *AIDS Education and Prevention, 16,* 405–414.

Jean, D., & Sen, A. (1995). *India: Economic Development and Social Opportunity,* Delhi: Oxford University Press.

John, T. J., Babu, P. G., Jayakumari, H., & Simoes, E. A. (1987). Prevalence of HIV infection among risk groups in Tamilnadu, India. *Lancet, 1,* 160–161.

Joint United Nations Programme on HIV/AIDS. (2004a). *India Epidemiological Fact Sheet—2004 Update.* Retrieved December 14, 2005, from http://www.who.int/GlobalAtlas/predefinedReports/EFS2004/EFS_PDFs/EFS2004_IN.pdf

Joint United Nations Programme on HIV/AIDS. (2004b). *2004 Report on the global AIDS epidemic—Table of country-specific HIV/AIDS estimates and data, end 2003.* Retrieved December 14, 2005, from http://www.unaids.org/bangkok2004/report_pdf.html

Joint United Nations Programme on HIV/AIDS. (2005a). *AIDS epidemic update: December 2005.* Retrieved December 14, 2005, from http://www.unaids.org/Epi2005/doc/report_pdf.html

Joint United Nations Programme on HIV/AIDS. (2005b). *India*. Retrieved December 12, 2005, from http://www.unaids.org/en/geographical+area/by+country/india.asp
Joint United Nations Programme on HIV/AIDS. (2006). *2006 Report on the global AIDS epidemic*. Retrieved July 24, 2006, from http://www.unaids.org/en/HIV_data/2006GlobalReport/default.asp
Kumar, R., Jha, P., Arora, P., Mony, P., Bhatia, P., Millson, P., et al. (2006). Trends in HIV-1 in young adults in south India from 2000 to 2004: A prevalence study. *Lancet, 367*, 1164–1172.
Manjunath, J. V., Thappa, D. M., & Jaisankar, T. J. (2002). Sexually transmitted diseases and sexual lifestyles of long-distance truck drivers: A clinico-epidemiologic study in south India [Electronic version]. *International Journal of STD & AIDS, 13*, 612–617.
Mehendale, S. M., Shepherd, M. E., & Divekar, A. D. (1996). Evidence for high prevalence and rapid transmission of HIV among individuals attending STD clinics in Pune, India. *Indian Journal of Medical Research, 104*, 327–335.
Menen-Sen, K., & Shiva Kumar, A. K. (2001). *Women in India: How Free? How Equal?* Retrieved December 12, 2005 from United Nations Web site http://www.un.org.in/wii.htm
Menon, R. (2004). *Tomorrow's citizens: Imperiled today*. Retrieved December 15, 2005 from India Together Web site http://www.indiatogether.org/2004/nov/chi-hazards.htm
Merchant, R. H., & Lala, M. M. (2005). Prevention of mother-to-child transmission of HIV-an overview [Electronic version]. *Indian Journal of Medical Research, 121*, 489–501.
Nagelkerke, N. J. D., Jha, P., de Vlas, S. J., Korenromp, E. L., Moses, S., Blanchard, J. F., et al. (2002). Modelling HIV/AIDS epidemics in Botswana and India: Impact of interventions to prevent transmission [Electronic version]. *Bulletin of the World health Organization, 80*, 89–96.
National AIDS Control Organization (NACO). (2004a). *National guidelines for implementation of antiretroviral therapy (ART)*. Retrieved December 15, 2005, from http://www.nacoonline.org/guidelines/ART_Guidelines.pdf
National AIDS Control Organization (NACO). (2004b). *Annual Report 2002–2003, 2003–2004 (up to 31 July, 2004)*. Retrieved April 3, 2006, from http://www.nacoonline.org/annualreport/annulareport.pdf
National AIDS Control Organization (NACO). (2005a). *Monthly updates on AIDS (31 July, 2005)*. Retrieved December 14, 2005, from http://www.nacoonline.org/facts_report july.htm
National AIDS Control Organization (NACO). (2005b). *An overview of the spread and prevalence of HIV/AIDS in India*. Retrieved December 14, 2005, from http://www.nacoonline.org/facts_overview.htm
National AIDS Control Organization (NACO). (2005c). *Observed HIV prevalence levels state wise: 1998-2004*. Retrieved December 14, 2005, from http://www.nacoonline.org/facts_statewise.htm
National AIDS Control Organization (NACO). (2005d). *HIV estimates-2004*. Retrieved December 14, 2005, from http://www.nacoonline.org/facts_hivestimates04.htm

National AIDS Control Organization (NACO). (2005e). *Directory of Services—Statewise list of NGOs*. Retrieved December 15, 2005, from http://www.nacoon line.org/directory_ngo.htm

Panda, S., Chatterjee, A., Bhattacharya, S. K., Manna, B., Singh, P. N., Sarkar, S., et al. (2000). Transmission of HIV from injecting drug users to their wives in India [Electronic version]. *International Journal of STD & AIDS, 11*, 468–473.

Population Communications International. (2005). *Fighting HIV/AIDS: From family tragedies to social upheaval*. Retrieved November 30, 2005 from http://www. population.org/thematic_fightinghivaids.shtml

Risbud, A. (2005). Human immunodeficiency virus (HIV) and sexually transmitted diseases (STDs) [Electronic version]. *Indian Journal of Medical Research, 121,* 369–376.

Rodrigues, J. J., Mehendale, S. M., & Shepherd, M. E. (1995). Risk factors for HIV infection in people attending clinics for sexually transmitted diseases in India. *British Medical Journal, 311,* 283–286.

Self Employed Women's Association. (2005). *Campaigns*. Retrieved December 12, 2005 from http://sewa.org/campaigns/index.htm

Sharma, D. C. (2000). India challenges UN agencies' estimates of HIV prevalence [Electronic version]. *Lancet, 356,* 662.

Simoes, E. A., Babu, P. G., John, T. J., Nirmala, S., Solomon, S., Lakshinarayana, C. S., et al. (1987). Evidence for HTLV-III infection in prostitutes in Tamil Nadu (India). *Indian Journal of Medical Research, 85,* 335–338.

Solomon, S., Chakraborty, A., & Yepthomi, R. D. (2004). A review of the HIV epidemic in India [Electronic version]. *AIDS Education and Prevention, 16*(Supp A), 155–169.

Thukral, E. J. Poverty and gender in India: Issues for concern. *Proceedings from First Asia and Pacific Forum on Poverty*. Retrieved December 12, 2005, from http://www.adb.org/Documents/Books/Defining_Agenda_ Poverty_Reduction/Vol_1/chapter_23.pdf

Ukey, P. M., Akulwar, S. L., & Powar, R. M. (2005). Seroprevalence of human immunodeficiency virus infection in pregnancy in a tertiary care hospital [Electronic version]. *Indian Journal of Medical Sciences, 59,* 382–387.

U.N. official doubts India on AIDS data. (2005, November 21). *New York Times*. Retrieved December 14, 2005, from http://www.nytimes.com

United States Agency for International Development. (2005). *Strategic objective 5: Enhanced opportunities for vulnerable people*. Retrieved April 6, 2006, from http://www.usaid.gov/in/our_work/strategy/strategy8.htm

United States National Intelligence Council. (2002). *The next wave of HIV/ AIDS: Nigeria, Ethiopia, Russia, India, and China*. Retrieved December 14, 2005, from http://www.cia.gov/nic/PDF_GIF_otherprod/HIVAIDS/ICA_HIV AIDS20092302.pdf

Verma, R. K. & Collumbien, M. (2004). Homosexual activity among rural Indian men: Implications for HIV interventions [Electronic version]. *AIDS, 18,* 1845–1847.

World Bank. (2003, July 2). *Project performance assessment report: India, national AIDS control project*. Retrieved December 14, 2005, from http://www-wds.

worldbank.org/servlet/WDS_IBank_Servlet?pcont=details&eid=000094946_030 82104011041

World Bank. (2004). *Issue brief-poverty in India.* Retrieved December 14, 2005 from http://siteresources.worldbank.org/INTINDIA/Data%20and%20Reference/ 20283013/Poverty_India_Brief.pdf

World Health Organization. (2005). *The world health report 2005—make every mother and child count.* Retrieved December 14, 2005, from http://www.who. int/whr/2005/whr2005_en.pdf

Zaheer, K. (2005). India's HIV cases higher than official numbers. *Boston Globe.* Retrieved November 20, 2005, from http://www.boston.com/news/world/asia/articles/ 2005/11/20/indias_hiv_cases_higher_than_official_numbers/

Index

Printed in the United States
by Baker & Taylor Publisher Services